natural living
body care

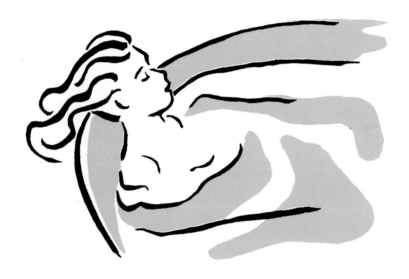

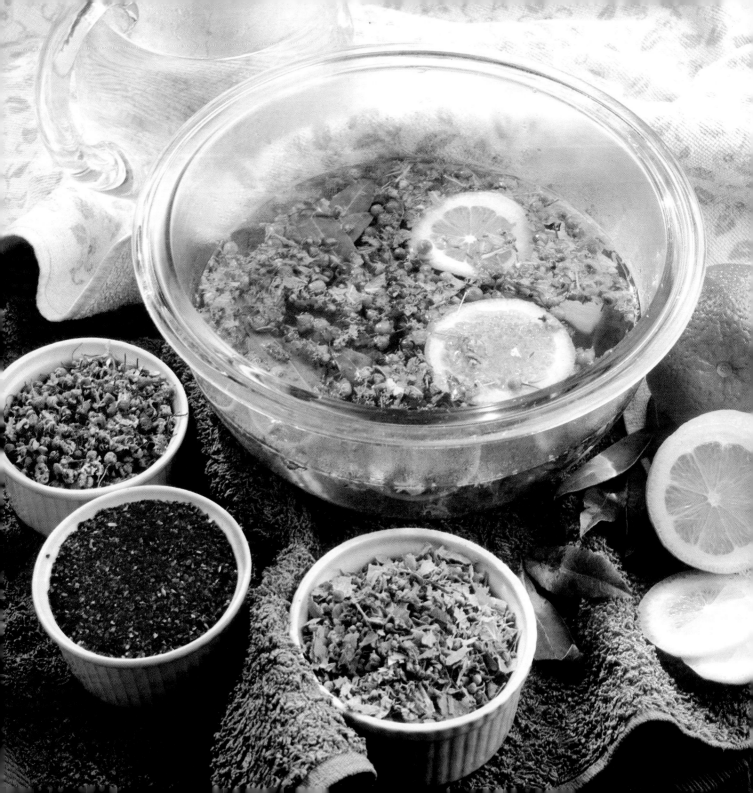

natural living
body care

Jennifer Powell

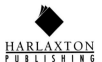

HARLAXTON
PUBLISHING

FRONT JACKET:
Fresh and natural body care preparations are easy to make. They contain no artificial ingredients. Enjoy pure and natural treatments at your leisure in your own home.

PAGE 2:
Rosehip facial sauna is quick to make and an excellent way to cleanse your skin. You can use it in the bath or just tie it up in several layers of muslin (cheesecloth).

Measurements
All spoon measurements are level.
As the imperial/metric/US equivalents are not exact, follow only one system of measurement.
Ovens should be preheated to the specified temperature.

Ingredients
Fresh herbs are used unless otherwise stated. If they are unavailable, use half the quantity of dried herbs.

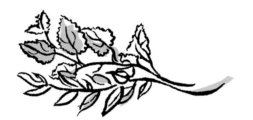

Published by Harlaxton Publishing Limited
2 Avenue Road, Grantham, NG31 6TA, United Kingdom
A Member of The Weldon International Group of Companies

First published 1994
© 1994 Copyright Harlaxton Publishing Ltd
© 1994 Copyright design Harlaxton Publishing Ltd

Publishing Manager: Robin Burgess
Project Coordinator: Barbara Beckett
Designer: Amanda McPaul
Illustrations: Kate Finnie
Photographers: Jill White and Ray Jarratt
Typesetting: Sellers, Grantham
Reproduction: G A Graphics, Stamford
Printing: Imago, Singapore

British Library Cataloguing-in-Publication data
A catalogue record for this book is available from the British Library
ISBN: 1-85837-061-2

Acknowledgements
Tony Stone Worldwide Photolibrary – pages 15, 35, 50, 57
Britstock-IFA Ltd – pages 33, 43

We would like to thank the models Emma Garrett and Sarah Crowe, for taking part in this book

Contents

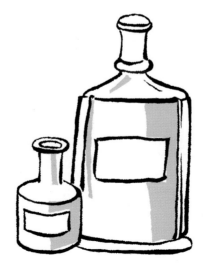

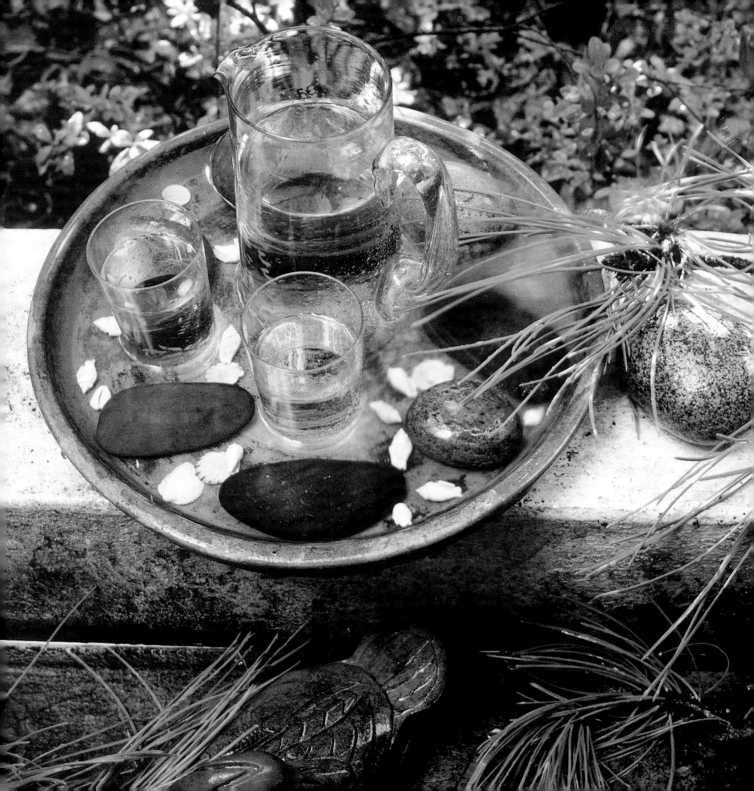

Introduction

Your body is working for you whether you are asleep or awake. Internal cleansing, healing and disease-fighting activities are continually occurring, so that you can function in a clean and healthy fashion and be restored to your natural beauty. Your body's hygiene and immune systems need special assistance in the more polluted and artificial environments of today.

Body care means looking after yourself from head to toe by understanding natural hygiene and using simple, natural preparations and remedies. There are so many advantages! Natural treatments are cheap, easy and fun to do at home. They are pure and fresh, with plenty of vitamins and minerals and no preservatives or drugs. You can tailor them to your own needs or tastes for use at times that suit you. They are 'environmentally friendly', involving no manufacturing, packaging or transport costs to you or the environment and avoid any testing on animals. Make bodycare products in your own home and luxuriate in natural treatments to keep you looking great.

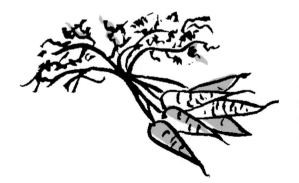

OPPOSITE:
It is cheap and easy to purify your water at home. Always use pure water for our recipes as well as to drink. Remember that the body needs six to eight glasses of water a day to aid its hygiene system.

Natural Hygiene

*T*he idea of body care evokes images of languishing in nourishing baths, enjoying deep massage and pedicures. It also rests on a good understanding of your own private hygiene system – how does your body rejuvenate itself, get rid of poisonous wastes or find its own flexible equilibrium midst the toil and stress of modern life? How can you keep your body healthy and feeling good, beautiful and responsive to all the demands you place upon it?

D amaging environmental conditions place a harsh burden on your skin. Air conditioning and central heating add another toll. Greater stress in modern life and higher levels of chemicals in food, water and air give your cleansing, immune and waste disposal systems a tough time.

There are plenty of expensive treatments available. What you really need, however, are simple, natural, everyday routines that keep you looking good. You also need to learn the small signs that indicate action is required. You are unique. You can use nature and nature's products – water and sunshine, fragrant herbs and natural oils, fresh fruit and vegetables all provide the ingredients for healthy life-giving body treatments. You can whip up simple remedies in response to the slightest changes!

How the body cleanses itself

T he body is engaged in constant cleansing. Waste products from food digestion and metabolism must be removed. These waste products include heat, carbon dioxide, water, solid waste, minerals and urea (from the breakdown of protein). Old cells, pollutants, foreign bodies and harmful micro-organisms are dealt with too. The body recycles what it requires, as it cleanses itself in a continuous cyclical process to maintain optimum hygiene and health.

Heat, water and carbon dioxide are lost through the skin and lungs. The skin also excretes some salts and urea through perspiration. The kidneys dispense with urea, minerals and some toxins. The lymphatic and blood systems carry out the major role of fighting disease as well as removing old cells and harmful pollutants. The lymphatic system influences how our body looks and feels – it concentrates on body fluids around the cells.

The lymphatic system

A lthough most people know little about their lymphatic system – except when their glands or lymph nodes swell up – it is an essential part of our immune or disease-fighting apparatus – without it we could not live!

OPPOSITE:
Herbal baths are easy to make and give you a tremendous lift. Anyone in the vicinity of the bathroom benefits as wonderful fragrances permeate the house!

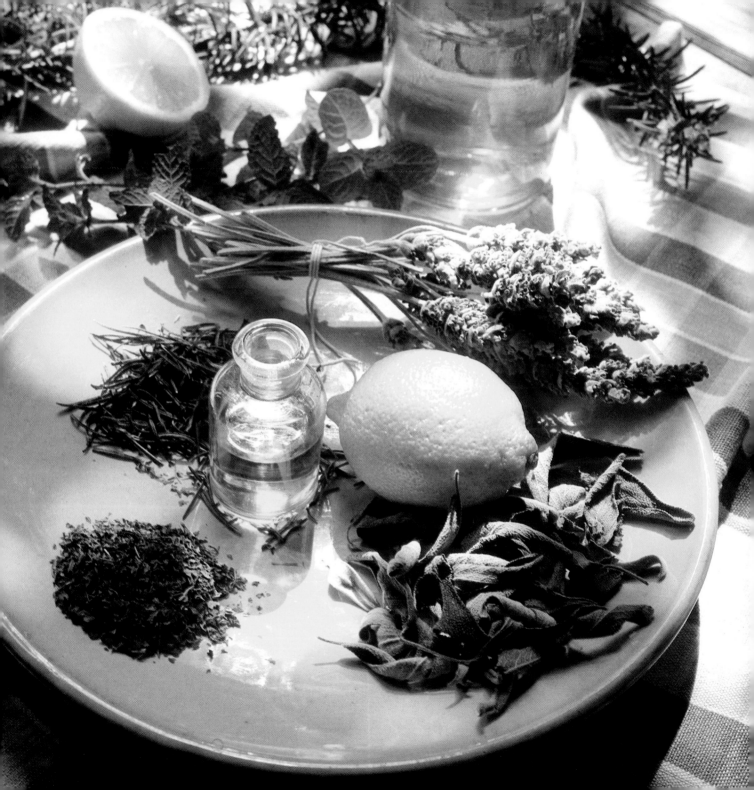

THE LYMPHATIC SYSTEM:
Tiny lymph vessels follow our
blood system all over the body
draining off poisons and wastes.
At intervals, lymph nodes deal
with them, sometimes becoming
quite painful and swollen when
infection is spreading. Plenty of
water, exercise and rest aid their
work as does a good diet.

1   *Lymph nodes*
2   *Large lymph ducts*
3   *Lymph capillaries*

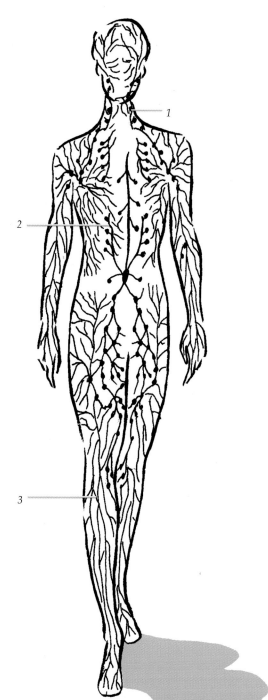

All the cells in the body are bathed in a watery fluid called lymph. Tiny lymph capillaries (very thin tubes) renew the lymph and monitor it, draining off waste material, dead cells and disease-causing micro-organisms from around the cells. These are carried in the lymph capillaries into large ducts that eventually empty into a channel along the spine. At intervals, lymph nodes control the flow of this fluid and stop disease spreading by destroying micro-organisms and toxins. When these nodes become swollen you know that they are busy at work. There are many lymph nodes in the neck, under the arms, near the liver and intestines and in the groin. Eventually, after cleansing, the lymph fluid returns to the bloodstream.

Fighting disease

The skin is usually the first line of defence against germs entering the body. Millions of germs can live on the skin quite harmlessly – provided they go no further. When we become run down, however, they can multiply faster, spread deeper and cause illness. Saliva, tears and stomach juices kill many attacking bacteria and viruses. Once they reach the inner parts of the body, however, the lymphatic and blood systems must take over the battle.

Lymph nodes produce special white cells which engulf harmful bacteria, digesting them. Some germs have protective coats which cannot be digested by white cells unless they are punctured first. Both the lymph and blood contain vast armies of different antibodies which react with foreign protein on the surface of the invading micro-organisms, puncturing or altering their protective coats so that the white cells can dispose of them. Antibodies are produced in the lymph nodes, spleen or elsewhere, in response to each type of micro-organism entering the body fluids. This is how vaccines work, by causing the body to manufacture specific antibodies. Once

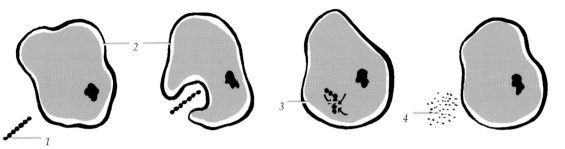

WHITE CELLS DESTROYING A
HARMFUL MICRO-ORGANISM:
*A white cell approaches and
surrounds an invading micro-
organism. Chemicals inside the
cell destroy the germ, digesting it.*

1   Micro-organism (germ)
2   White cell
3   Micro-organism being
      digested
4   Waste

antibodies are made, they remain in the body for some time, ready for action.

Removing wastes and poisons

Every metabolic reaction in the body involves the production of waste or leftover chemicals which may be harmful if allowed to build up in the tissues and body fluids. In addition, increasing pollution in our air, water and food add to the toxic substances that must be constantly cleansed from our blood and cells for effective operation. At the same time, millions of cells are dying and being replaced by new ones. Dead cells must be dismantled and removed, and appropriately recycled. When cells are injured, they must be broken down and carried away with any excess fluid, before new cells can be built to replace the damaged tissues. Fibrous traps in the lymph nodes filter the fluid and neutralize all harmful substances.

There is no pump to move the lymph through the body. It is only pressure from breathing, from muscle movement and from surrounding tissues that can actually squeeze the lymph along. Hence, exercise and good muscle tone are very important to stimulate the flow of lymph, while relaxation releases blockages and tension to allow the efficient removal of wastes. Massage also assists lymph movement. A clogged, swollen lymph system can be eased by some of the techniques we discuss in this book. Much water therapy is based on either relaxing blocked lymph or stimulating movement of sluggish lymph, depending on the condition.

The water balance in your body is crucial to all chemical processes. You consist of approximately 60 per cent water by weight. Water is required to detoxify your body from harmful bacteria and the modern poisons we live among, as well as to remove metabolic wastes and dead cells. Cleansing processes that occur in the kidneys, for example, or in the lymph system also require energy and a complex battery of enzymes to work well. A highly nutritious diet with the right balance of minerals and plenty of fluid are essential components of natural hygiene and a healthy immune system. Healthy skin and muscle tone also play their role.

The skin

To encourage the good skin that we all want, it helps to understand how it works. The skin is considered a body organ because it actively performs so many functions. First, it is a tough, protective, self-replacing layer that is waterproof and guards the

tip

Did you know that a range of harmless bacteria live on the skin? No matter how vigorously we scrub ourselves, some of these full-time residents will remain. Some in fact protect us from more harmful bacteria which can penetrate damaged skin and cause infections. Immediate cleansing with antiseptic remedies – eucalyptus, tea-tree, thyme – will stop them in their tracks!

THE SKIN:

Our skin has so many tiny organs just under the surface. As well as being a protective layer, it helps to regulate temperature and water and relays signals from the outside world!

1   Hair
2   Sensory receptor
3   Oil gland
4   Hair follicle
5   Sweat gland
6   Blood vessel
7   Pore
8   Epidermis
9   Dermis

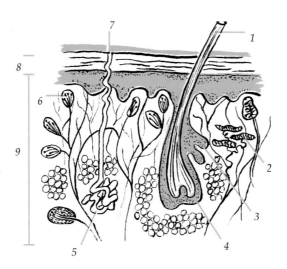

OPPOSITE:

The skin ages naturally but, of course, most of us would like to slow down the process! Vital and glowing skin is best maintained by using natural preparations and treatments that allow the skin to follow its own rhythms.

body against injury, attack from harmful micro-organisms and other environmental hazards. Its complex system of nerve sensors alert you to touch, temperature and pressure changes and other warning signals. It is the body's most important means of cooling itself, because heat can be quickly dispersed through myriads of tiny blood vessels near the surface, and through sweat-gland pores.

There are two basic layers of the skin, which is a highly complex structure. The outer layer, or epidermis, is very densely packed with cells. New cells are constantly being produced at the base and rising to the surface where they die, forming a hard protective layer. Millions of these dead cells are worn or washed away from the skin each day.

The second layer is called the dermis and is much stronger, thicker and more elastic, providing the blood supplies to produce epidermal cells and being richly endowed with many nerves connected to the receptors we need for sensations of pain, touch, cold or warmth. Hairs, sweat glands and oil glands grow in this layer and poke out through the epidermis.

The oil glands release sebum, an oil, on to the skin, helping to keep the skin supple (your personal moisturizer) and, by absorbing some of the sunlight, assist in reducing sunburn. The skin is able to absorb UV radiation and use it to convert certain substances into vitamin D which you need for your body to absorb calcium properly. Sunshine also acts as a very efficient antibiotic. Too little sunlight can be as bad as too much!

The sweat glands are very important for both temperature regulation and removing wastes. Sometimes perspiration has an offensive smell either because of the diet or from certain bacteria that thrive in moist, warm conditions. We are beginning to appreciate the problems caused by blocking their natural action with excessive use of deodorants, very heavy creams or synthetic clothes.

The skin must 'breathe' – perspiration performs a natural cleansing function. There are many ways of turning this into a pleasant experience. Natural scented oil can mean your body gives off a delicious fragrance. See our suggestions on page 33. The correct use of water and baths can help deal with excessive perspiration.

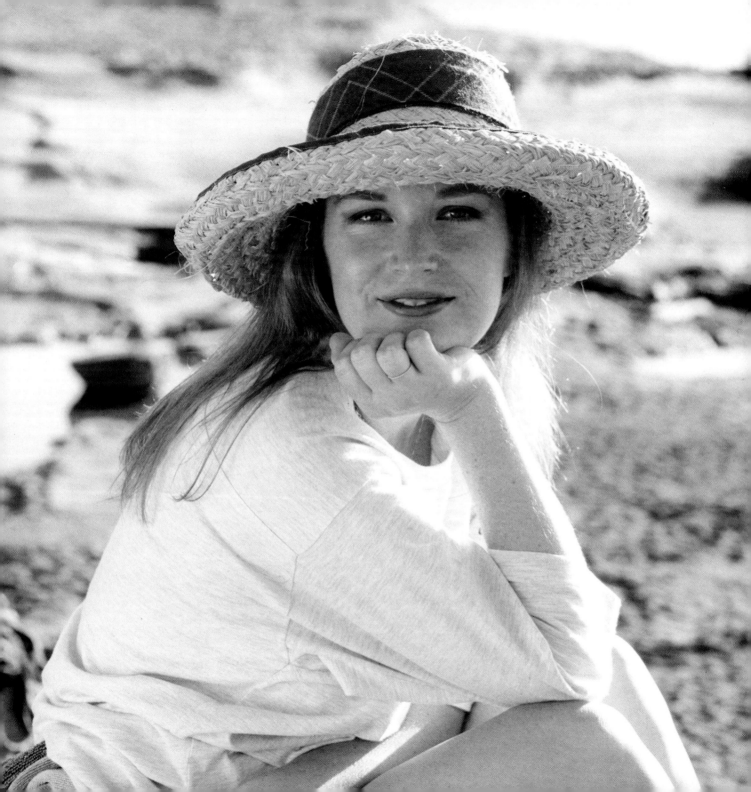

OPPOSITE:
A shower can be relaxing or revitalising. Control the force of the spray to give tired muscles a relaxing massage, or, try alternating the water temperature between warm and cold to leave you feeling refreshed and invigorated.

Water therapies

Water has wonderful healing qualities, either stimulating or soothing us depending on how we apply this gift from nature. It is often taken for granted, yet it can do so much for your health if you learn to rediscover some of the many simple treatments that were common in ancient times.

Essentially, water improves the skin, releasing wastes and old cells. It soothes the nervous system, including the brain and spine. It also aids blood flow and the work of the heart. By judicious use of temperature, it can ease pain and relax tired and stiff muscles. It is often overlooked as an everyday health remedy because it is so simple. The wise and creative use of water is an important aspect of body care.

Baths

One of the nicest and healthiest things you can do for yourself is to have a bath. Showers are good, but baths are even better. It is amazing the number of people who have lovely long bathtubs but rarely use them. Perhaps they have forgotten how good it feels. You can actually read and have a cup of tea in the bath – or listen to music!

Baths are particularly good for your natural hygiene system because of the time you spend in them. Soaking in water softens the outer skin layer far more than showering. A face cloth, loofah, massage glove or pumice stone will assist in the removal of dead skin. The skin pores will then be free to function really efficiently. A half-hour soak once a week is a health must and is beneficial if you are getting less sleep than usual. A bath can also speed up the natural cleansing process that normally occurs during sleep.

Another wonderful feature of baths is what you can put in them. You can add toners, like the herbal bath recipe on page 32, that will refresh and contract the skin, stimulating circulation. Sea salt will act as a disinfectant and skin relaxer, as well as a skin tonic. Traditional Epsom salts soothe the muscles and are well known as a sports remedy after exhausting physical exercise. Moisturizers and oils can also be added to improve your skin.

You can treat yourself with aromatherapy in a bath. Popular aromatherapy oils (often called essential oils) include lavender, which is relaxing, and camomile, which also heals the skin. Thyme oil will act as a tonic and rosemary oil is said to aid sleep. What delicious scents will issue from the bathroom! Be sure to add only a few drops to the water, as aromatherapy oils are quite concentrated. See page 21 for aromatherapy oils.

Showers

One of the chief benefits of the simple shower is its capacity to work muscles gently as you control the force of the spray, and massage yourself. Water temperature can be altered very quickly too and you can give yourself a quick taste of hydrotherapy. First, use warm water to stimulate blood flow to the skin, relax muscles and open the pores that get rid of wastes. Then a brief change to cold water will contract the skin, tone the muscles and send the blood away again. This will close the pores to stop water loss, but can leave you feeling too cold, so ensure you do not use cold water for too long – 30 to 60 seconds only. Repeat this a couple of times and your whole body will surge with energy. This is a simple technique to give yourself a big lift if you have not had enough sleep or exercise.

Facial steams and saunas

Cleansing your face regularly with aromatic, steaming water assists your skin to rid itself of impurities. The water molecules actively accelerate the cleansing process by stimulating perspiration.

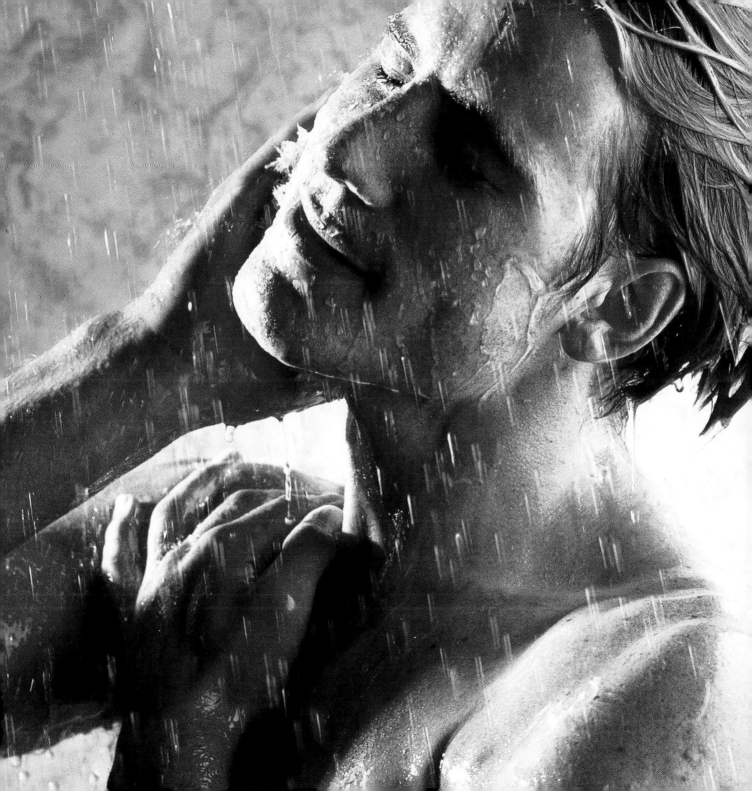

This releases wastes and dirt from the pores along with any old make-up and creams that may have lodged more deeply in the skin.

The blood flow increases, enhancing the production of new cells, and aiding the removal of excess dead ones. Any fragrant herbs or oils you may add to the water can have further beneficial effects, depending on your own particular needs. For example, camomile oil is soothing and thyme more cleansing. Refer to our Aromatherapy table on page 21 for inspiration. There are two special facial sauna recipes on pages 26 and 28.

Before preparing your facial steam, remove all make-up. Put 1 tablespoon dried herbs of your choice or 10 drops aromatherapy oil into a large ceramic bowl. Pour in enough boiling water at least to half-fill the bowl. Cover your head with a towel to trap steam on to your face, checking it is not too hot. Only steam for 5 minutes. Avoid this technique if your skin is sensitive, dry or broken, or if you suffer from asthma or a heart condition.

Inhalations

Inhalations can be prepared in the same way as facial steams and are extremely useful for clearing the respiratory tract of mucus – for colds, blocked sinuses and coughs. Use appropriate aromatherapy and antiseptic oils such as eucalyptus, thyme, peppermint, cajeput or tea-tree. Remember to breathe in deeply through the nose, and alternate from nostril to nostril if very heavily blocked. It works gradually. Inhalations can be repeated three times a day for serious congestion. These are beneficial if used before going to sleep.

Foot baths

Relax your feet (or hands) in a bowl of fragrant, hand-hot water while sitting down in the evenings. Keep some extra hot water handy in a kettle to add as the water cools. Ten to 15 minutes is long enough. Move your feet or hands occasionally. After soaking, wrap them up in a dry towel for another 10 minutes. Finish off with a little massage that includes the lower legs. Aromatherapy oils can be added to both the bath and the massage oil.

Compresses and sitz baths

Both compresses and sitz baths are old-fashioned remedies and many of the particular skills required have almost been lost to us. Fortunately, they are being rediscovered and health spas often use these healing treatments. They were once used extensively for feminine ailments such as painful periods. Experiment with simpler techniques to assist skin and muscular problems, and headaches.

The ice compress is still used for burns, bruises and other tissue injury to reduce swelling caused by the initial shock and cell damage. However, where there is a long-term injury or complaint that requires regular treatment over a period of time, it is important to consult someone experienced in these treatments, especially if you have serious circulatory or heart problems. This is because of the alternate use of hot and cold water. We hope that, with time, the therapeutic value of these techniques will be explored thoroughly and adequate safeguards established so we can all have access once again to their benefits.

COMPRESSES – are usually pieces of cotton, soaked in hot, warm or cold water (often containing some aromatherapy oils) that are placed over the problem area to stimulate healing. A cold-water compress over the forehead and another at the back of the neck is good for a headache. Lavender and sage oils work well. An especially severe headache will benefit from a hot foot bath at the same time! Painful periods can be eased by placing a cold compress covered with a towel over the lower abdomen. Leave for 10

tip

Add an aromatic flavour to your shower! Smooth massage oil containing essential oil over your body, then shower. You can even keep the plug in, adding a few drops to the water. As the aroma arises, you benefit from wonderful herbal vapours. Try peppermint, rosemary or lemon grass to uplift your day!

minutes to relieve congestion – a very old technique. Hot-water compresses are very good for painful joints and muscles. Eucalyptus and rosemary oils can be added. Eye compresses relieve sore or tired eyes. See page 42.

SITZ BATHS – are more complicated in that you require two large bowls, one of warm and one of cool water. You alternate by sitting in the warm water, with the feet in the cool water and then swapping over at frequent intervals. This increases blood flow into the entire pelvic area as well as toning delicate muscles, so that congestion and impurities are removed, and additional healing comes with extra fresh blood. Recommended timings vary considerably and require further research as each condition would need a different treatment. The best idea is to go to a health clinic or spa where experienced staff will design a sitz bath regimen to suit your personal requirements.

Water temperature

Alternating hot/warm and cold water is an important tool in water therapies. Hot water expands blood vessels, relaxes muscles and opens skin pores, releasing water and wastes. This stimulates cell activity by drawing an extra volume of warm, fresh blood to the area. Cold water causes blood vessels to compress and sweat glands to close, tones the muscles and impels the blood deeper into the body. It is only applied for a short period – the body responds by rapidly sending more fresh nutrient-rich blood to the area.

Temperatures in baths can also be varied subtly. A warm bath relaxes muscles and relieves fatigue and pain. A cooler bath, however, is more soothing and assists sleep. This was once used to calm agitated mental patients!

NOTE: Never use alternating hot and cold water treatments on babies, the elderly or anyone with heart problems.

INHALATIONS:

Inhalations remove nasal and head congestion using steam and eucalyptus oil. Many water treatments are simple, old-fashioned remedies that have been used in different cultures for centuries.

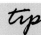

tip

Spas are built in wonderful places where nature's mineral waters rise to the surface for us to use in hydropathy – drinking, or bathing, steaming or soaking in these health-giving waters has great therapeutic value. Seawater therapy is available too – antiseptic salt water cleanses the skin, nose, ears and eyes. Traditional in Europe, spas are now appearing in many other countries around the world.

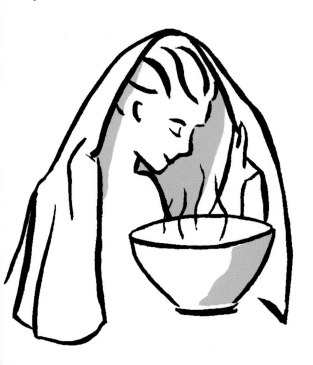

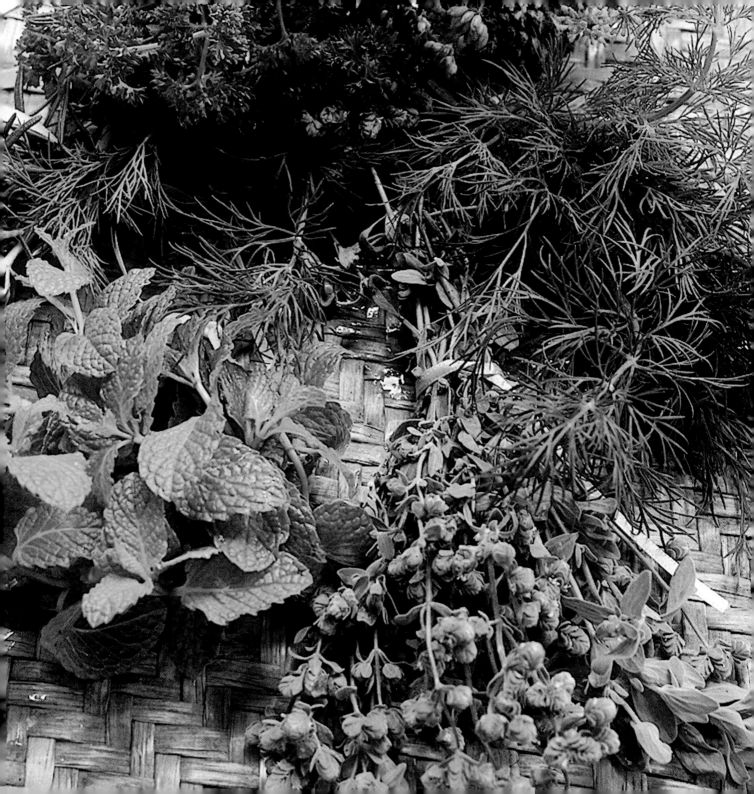

Aromatic Herbs

When natural body care and healing are mentioned, nothing springs to mind more clearly than the beauty and wealth of the aromatic herbs. Often modest in size, the potency of their oil quite offsets their appearance. Down the ages they have adorned the lives of many peoples in a variety of ways.

Aromatic herbs are used for simple pleasure in food and perfumes, or as healing agents. The art of using the scent of herbs in healing is now known as aromatherapy. Other parts of herbs are used in remedies as well – the seeds, bark, roots, flowers and leaves are all of value.

Healing qualities

The healing value of herbs lies in the way they concentrate vitamins, minerals and essential oils. Vitamins and minerals are indispensable for most bodily processes – we need continuous supplies of them. We know less about the precise benefit of the essential oils which contain the scent, although there is much information accumulating as modern science and natural therapies combine their efforts.

Tea-tree oil has proved to be a superb antibiotic in trials with harmful micro-organisms but precise responses to every scent are not so easy to measure. The psychological effects of fragrances are taken for granted, yet understanding how they work is another matter. Olfaction, or the sense of smell, is linked to the brain, the nervous and hormonal systems which in turn affect physiology, how organs work and how we feel. Researchers are just beginning to explore what herbs do as well as how they do it.

Generally aromatic herbs are reputed to have tremendous physical, emotional and mental benefits. Their reputation is based on thousands of years of human experience in a variety of cultures, so it seems there is something of great value to explore.

The active healing properties of the aromatic herbs are absorbed into the body in a number of ways – through the skin in a massage oil, through the nose and lungs as a scent or inhalation, and through our digestion in a tea or added to food.

Some simple suggestions

When choosing and assessing different herbs and oils to use, decide whether you want a soothing or stimulating effect, an antiseptic or uplifting quality. Camomile, for example, is gentle and soothing as a tea, while rosemary is strongly flavoured and vibrant in cooking. Bear in mind that herbal lore was and still is a complex and subtle discipline. Begin simply and modestly with widely favoured aromatic herbs – those with an excellent reputation! Our Aromatherapy table on page 21 has been constructed in this fashion. Some of the rarer herbs and oils can be more difficult to find. Collecting herbs can be a rewarding pastime as you continue your explorations over the years.

General properties

Aromatic herbs offer a wonderful range of natural hygienic properties. They are antiseptic, often able to kill off bacteria and fungi that invade the skin and body. Tea-tree oil is a powerful antibiotic,

OPPOSITE:
Herbs are noted for their delicate leaf architecture and for the wide variety in leaf shape and colour, as well as for their exquisite fragrances. When they flower, the new leaves are often quite different.

AROMATHERAPY OILS:
The strength and quality of aromatherapy oils depends on the method of extraction and how much vegetable oil they are mixed with. Incense oils are always more concentrated.

equivalent to many drugs, and both cinnamon and thyme oils have antiseptic properties. Some herbs are expectorants, encouraging the body to rid itself of excess mucus in the throat, nose and chest. Eucalyptus and sage oils are excellent expectorants, used directly on the skin or inhaled.

Other healing properties include the ability to act as astringents, cleansing and toning skin tissue so that the skin pores contract and the skin surface tightens up, thus improving defence against micro-organisms seeking to penetrate the surface. Witch hazel is the best known astringent. Many herbs act as stimulants, encouraging the blood flow to areas where extra nutrient-rich blood is required. One of the best known ointments is Chinese Tiger Balm which provides excellent relief for muscular pain, and contains camphor oil. Both rosemary and lemon oil are stimulating too.

A range of herbs act as soothing relaxants, encouraging the body to slow down over-stimulated nervous activity and release emotional tension so that its own healing processes can occur more efficiently and steadily. Valerian and camomile are both noted for this, valerian in particular being a well-respected cure for insomnia. Herbs that are uplifting and refreshing in effect are a wonderful boon in modern life – easing emotions, inspiring fresh ideas. Rose, amber, bergamot, neroli, frankincense, lavender, geranium and sandalwood are a few of the many delightful fragrances that may be subtle and yet act as a powerful positive influence.

Herbs are some of the most rewarding plants to grow and savour. If you are lucky, you can grow your own and have the added delight of harvesting, drying and preparing them at home. Remember to give our preparations and remedies a fair trial. We have chosen very simple ones for you to begin with, as an introduction to aromatic herbs.

tip

Healthy soils mean healthy plants with plenty of vitamins and minerals for us to eat.
Be an environmentally friendly buyer where possible. Buy fresh, natural organic, biodynamic or free-range produce to support chemical-free agriculture. Buy local produce to reduce transport and storage costs. Refuse extra packaging and always recycle!

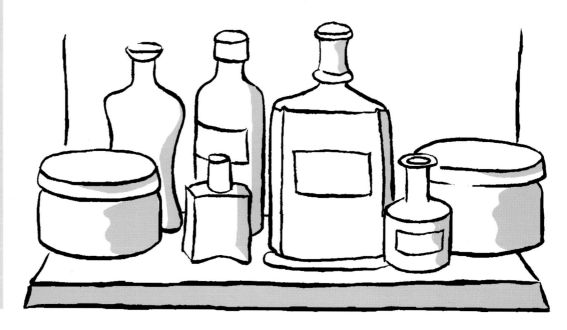

Aromatherapy

You will find a basic aromatherapy guide here and some preparation information. Specific suggestions on the use of herbs in home-made preparations and herbal teas may be found in other chapters.

Quantities of aromatherapy oils

Only very small quantities of essential oils are needed. General recommendations:

BATHS	5 to 10 drops
FOOT/HAND BATHS	5 to 10 drops for up to 3 litres/ 5¼ pints/3½ quarts water
COMPRESSES, SKIN TONICS	5 drops per 5½ table-spoons water
INHALATIONS, FACIAL STEAMS	10 drops in 600 ml/ 1 pint/2½ cups water
MASSAGE OILS	15 drops in 5½ table-spoons oil

Aromatherapy table

Oils	Qualities
AMBER	soothing, strengthening
BASIL	uplifting, clearing
BERGAMOT	uplifting, refreshing, relaxing
CAJEPUT	antiseptic, stimulating
CAMOMILE	relaxing
CAMPHOR	stimulating
CEDARWOOD	sedative, warming
CINNAMON	antiseptic
CLOVE	antiseptic
CYPRESS	toning, refreshing
EUCALYPTUS	decongestant, stimulating
FRANKINCENSE	relaxing, refreshing
GERANIUM	soothing, relaxing
JASMINE	relaxing, uplifting
JUNIPER	refreshing, easing
LAVENDER	uplifting, soothing
LEMON	refreshing, stimulating
LEMON GRASS	toning, relaxing
MARIGOLD	antiseptic
MARJORAM	warming
MUSK	fortifying
MYRRH	toning, releasing
NEROLI	uplifting
OREGANO	antiseptic, warming
PATCHOULI	relaxing
PEPPERMINT	soothing, refreshing
PINE	refreshing, antiseptic
ROSE	soothing, relaxing
ROSEMARY	stimulating, refreshing
SAGE	decongestant
SANDALWOOD	uplifting, relaxing
TANGERINE	gentle, soothing
TEA-TREE	excellent antiseptic
THYME	antiseptic
YLANG-YLANG	relaxing

tip

It is important to use pure, fresh products. Do not put anything on your skin to which you have an allergy. If in doubt, experiment with the mixture on the inside of your forearms – cover with a band-aid and leave for 24hrs.

NOTE: Essential oils are very potent and can easily be diluted with vegetable oil.

OPPOSITE:
*Rose-water is easy to make. Use
freshly gathered young rose petals.
As rose-water is used in cosmetics
and confectionery it can be bought
cheaply from specialist grocery
shops. See our recipe on this page.*

tip

*P*urify your water in your
own home. it is the simplest
way to be sure your drinking
and cooking water is chemical
free. For best results, always
use purified water, distilled
water or still mineral water in
our recipes.

Recipes

Buy your herbs, oils and incense at local health
food or specialist shops for highest quality. Buy
and keep them in tightly sealed containers and store
them in cool, dark places, as they will lose their
strength if exposed to air, heat or light. Ideally,
vegetable oils should be cold pressed as heating
destroys vitamins during processing. For best effect,
aromatherapy or essential oils should be as high
in quality as you can afford. Always buy very fresh,
high-quality fruit and vegetables.

Preparations with vegetable oils can deteriorate
chemically, so place them in dark jars and do not
make too much at once. Wheatgerm oil will help
preserve them so add a little to your mixture.
Sandalwood oil is a good 'fixative' to ensure fragrances
last and can be added in tiny amounts once mixed.
In general, it is best to make up home-made
preparations for immediate use, and only store
massage or perfume oils. Store in sealed jars in a cool
and dark place.

Hygienic techniques are important for home-
made preparations, as no preservatives are used
and ingredients are fresh or involve sensitive oils
that can either evaporate or deteriorate. Therefore,
everything you use must be spotlessly clean and
all containers sterilized first in boiling water. Never
use the same containers again without resterilizing.
Use enamel or stainless steel bowls and saucepans,
and glass jars and bottles for storage. In addition,
you will usually need wooden spoons, and muslin
(cheesecloth) or a stainless steel sieve for straining.

Herbal infusions

You can easily extract herbal essences yourself
by making infusions from fresh or dried herbs.
An infusion is a tea that has been allowed to sit or
'steep' for longer so that more herbal essences are
dissolved into the water. Do not boil the infusion
or essential oils will evaporate and precious vitamins
be lost. Make up fresh each time, as it will only
keep for 1–2 days in the refrigerator. Remember
that dried herbs are about four times as strong as
fresh ones and are even stronger when ground.

*1 teaspoon dried (3 tablespoons fresh) herbs per
250 ml/8 fl oz/1 cup pure water*

Bring water to boil in stainless steel saucepan.
Pour over herbs in cup or pot. Cover and leave
for 10 to 20 minutes. Strain and drink or use in
preparations. Will keep for 1 to 2 days in refrigerator.

Extracting essential oils

You can do this yourself by adding flowers to pure
cold-pressed olive oil. Pick flowers fresh and
either place whole flowers or petals only in the oil.
Blend briefly or mix well. Use a little more oil than
flowers. Store in tightly sealed jar and stand at room
temperature in a sunny position. Leave for 2 to 3
weeks, shaking daily. Strain and store oil in a bottle.
You can concentrate this oil by adding more flowers
and repeating.

Rose-water

To make your own rose-water, collect rose petals
early in the morning, place in an enamel pan and
just cover with pure water. Very slowly bring to
the boil and simmer for 4 minutes. Strain.

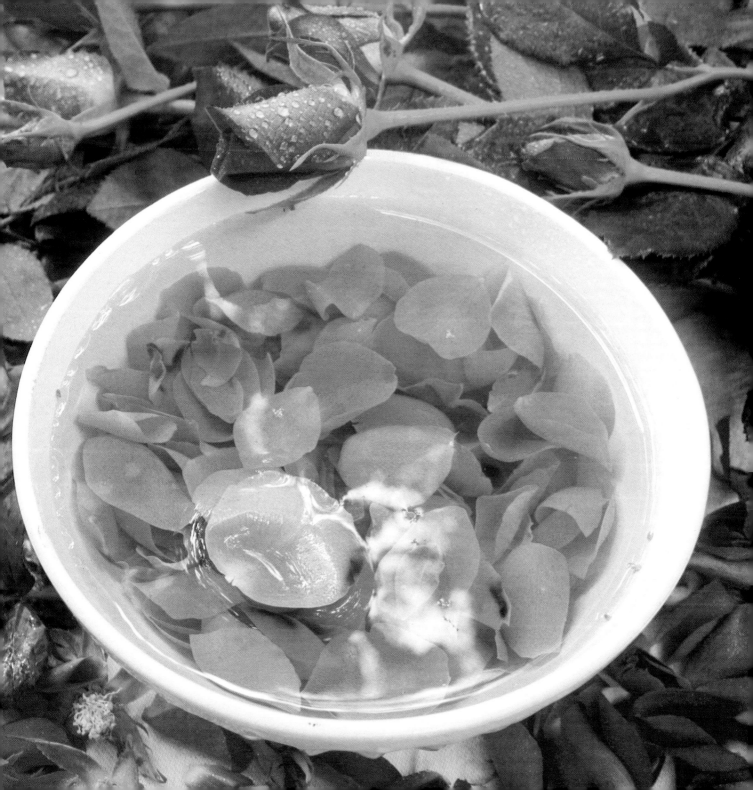

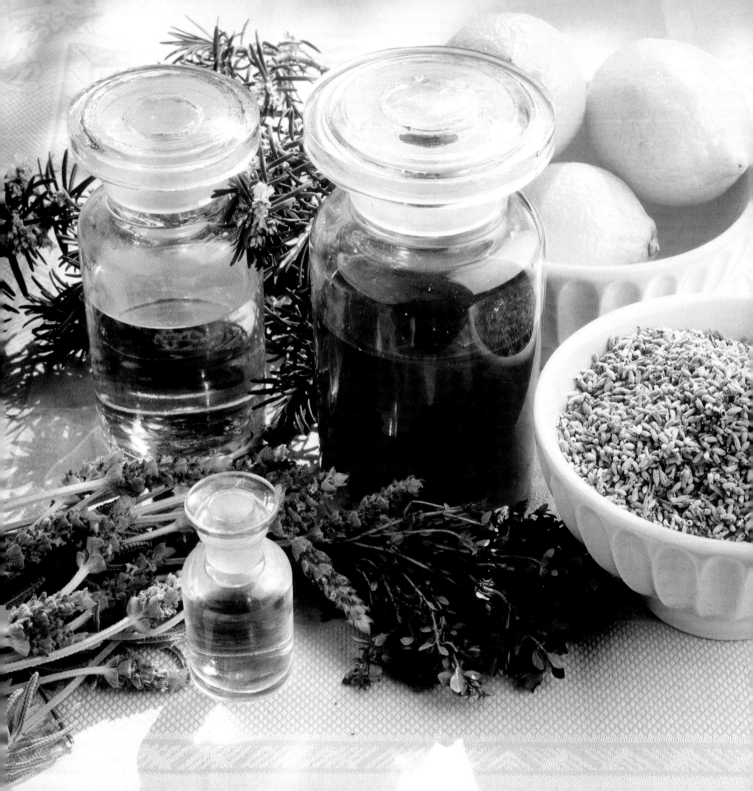

Skin and Hair Preparations

For a healthy, shining complexion and soft, resilient, yet firm body skin, natural products are the answer! They encourage the cleansing and disease-fighting properties of the skin while assisting it to renew and nourish itself constantly as surface layers wear out. If you remember that the skin is an important way to lose wastes and a protection from invading bacteria, you will find it easier to choose the right product for the right time.

It is no good putting on a heavy cream just before an intensive exercise workout that will certainly cause perspiration – especially when perspiring is one of the aims of the activity! It is better to apply a light protective oil on parts of the body that are exposed to the sun. Similarly, long soaks in warm, gently scented water will not help the skin if you have a fungal infection or badly dried-out skin. Epsom salts, bath oil, astringents and antiseptic essential oils will be more appropriate. So, remember that when you choose a skin treatment or protection, you need to cater to your own particular requirements with care.

The face

We are all conscious of our faces, and wish to keep the skin clear and healthy. It is also a highly sensitive and expressive area and you need to be responsive to all the changes that take place there. Exposed to temperature fluctuations, pollution and wear and tear by the elements, our facial skin is quick to signal when something is wrong.

As a general routine, cleanse the face to remove old make-up, dirt and dead cells. This tends to open the pores. Apply a toner to tighten the skin as well as re-establish the slightly acidic pH balance on the surface. Then moisturize to replace the natural oils and add extra nourishment.

Facial skin, like all skin, goes through various cycles of natural cleansing – for women it often follows the menstrual cycle. When blemishes occur, the normal routine can be suspended for a while and the face simply protected with a very light oil and only cleansed with cold water. This leaves it relatively free to correct the imbalance. By being flexible and observant we can respond to small changes as they appear. It is also important to avoid too much rubbing and scrubbing of facial skin which is only supported by delicate muscle and will easily stretch. Apply treatments and lotions by patting them on or massaging into the skin which will help stimulate its metabolic activity.

OPPOSITE:
Throughout history, herbs have been used in every culture to improve health, beauty and well-being. (We still have a lot to learn about this complex and fascinating discipline.) Lavender is one of the most popular and common ingredients in bodycare preparations.

tip

Instant face tonic – cut thin
slices of cucumber and gently
rub over your face, avoiding
the eye area. This will gently
tighten the skin tissue and
stimulate circulation, as well
as cleansing.

Recipes

Cleansers

You can cleanse your face every day with a light oil, a very mild vegetable-oil soap, milk, apple or grape juice or a cleanser! Oily skins will tend to produce more oil if too much soap is used. Diluted lemon juice will assist. A facial steam and / or a face mask once a week will cleanse thoroughly.

Rich face mask

1 egg
1 teaspoon honey
½ teaspoon brewers' yeast

Beat egg, mix with other ingredients. Smooth over wet face and leave for 15 minutes. Rinse off with warm water.

Apple face mask

Apple juice compress or application of pulped raw apple as a face mask tones tissue. Use muslin (cheesecloth) to hold the mask together if necessary. Apply to a wet face, leave 15 minutes and rinse off with warm water.

Milk and honey cleanser

2 teaspoons honey
2 tablespoons warm milk

Add honey to milk warming over a low heat. Blend well. Use your fingertips to massage this cleanser into your skin. Rinse off and pat your face dry with a towel.

Tropical fruit cleanser

This is very easy to make from the mineral-rich papaya (pawpaw) when it is in season. This is reputed to remove dead skin and give you an immediate lift.

30 g/1 oz/¼ cup mashed papaya (pawpaw)
1 teaspoon plain yoghurt

Mix ingredients and blend to a smooth paste. Gently pat the mixture on to your neck and face. Leave for 10 to 15 minutes then remove with warm water.

Herbal face steam

This treatment will cleanse your skin, stimulate circulation and leave you feeling fresh.

1 teaspoon dried parsley
1 teaspoon dried rosemary
1 teaspoon dried mint leaves
1 teaspoon dried marigold leaves
1 teaspoon dried camomile flowers
1.25 litres/2¼ pints/6 cups boiling water

First, cleanse your face of all make-up. Place all the herbs in the bottom of a bowl and carefully add the rapidly boiling water. After testing very carefully that the steam is not too hot, make a tent over your head and the bowl with a towel and steam your face for 5 minutes. Gently pat your face dry. If you like, follow with a mask and then close your pores with tepid water or a brisk skin tonic.

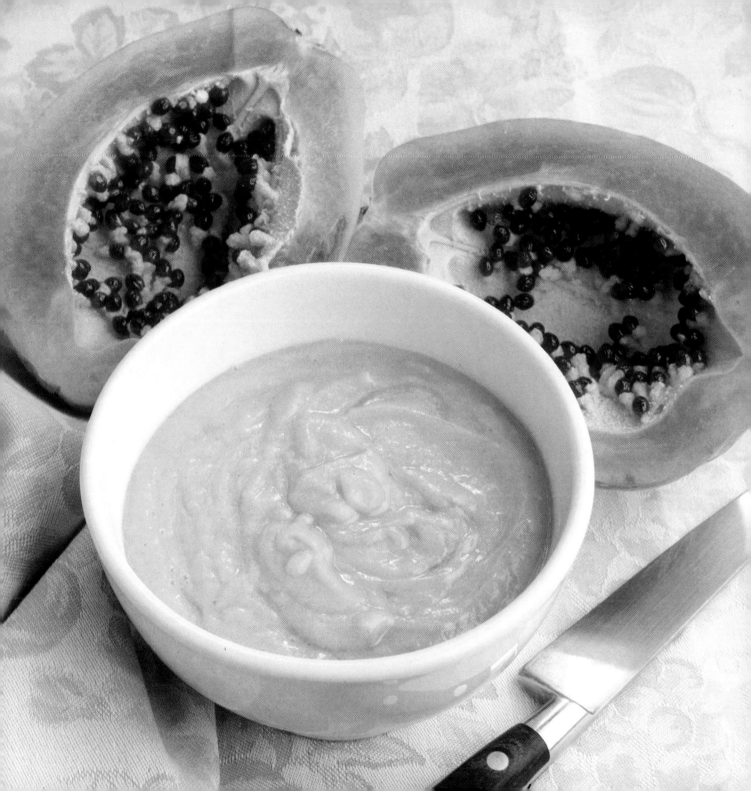

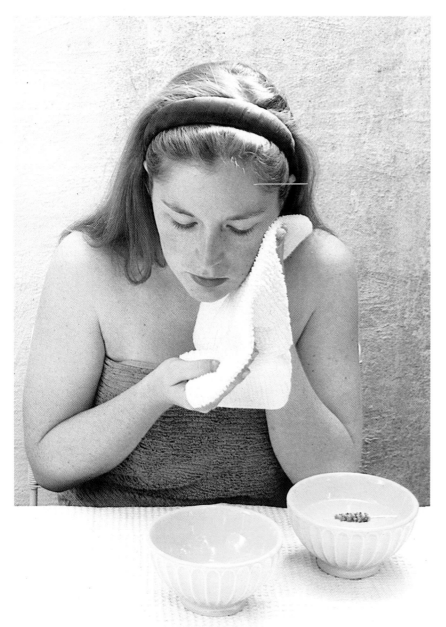

Rosehip facial sauna

1 teaspoon marjoram
1 teaspoon rosehips
1 teaspoon dried bay leaves
1 teaspoon camomile flowers
1 thin slice of lemon
1 thin slice of orange
1 teaspoon linden tea or flowers, optional
1.25 litres/2¼ pints/6 cups boiling water

Prepare as for previous recipe. This facial is very relaxing and soothing.

Toners

A simple toner for the face – add 1 teaspoon lemon juice to 2 tablespoons of pure water. Pat on, leave for 60 seconds and rinse off or leave, as preferred. Witch hazel, diluted with water, is an old favourite. Apply in the same way.

Herbal toners

1 teaspoon dried parsley
1 teaspoon fennel seeds
1 teaspoon camomile
600 ml/1 pint/2½ cups pure water
VARIATION
1 teaspoon peppermint
1 teaspoon thyme
1 teaspoon fennel seeds
600 ml/1pint/2½ cups pure water

Prepare an infusion as described on page 22. Either splash on or apply with cotton wool pads (swabs) to cleansed skin, then leave to dry.

Make up and try a sample of the variation as an alternative for spot or acne problems.

Vegetable toner

1 small, fresh cucumber
2 teaspoons strained lemon juice or witch hazel

Juice a fresh cucumber. Add 2 tablespoons to the lemon juice and shake well. Apply as above.

Moisturizers

Aloe vera gel by itself is a light moisturizer (add water for easier spreading). Pure, cold-pressed oils, including wheatgerm, avocado and olive oil, are also easy and rich moisturizers. Evening primrose oil can be used from the capsule for a luxury night oil or try the following, which are body moisturizers as well.

Aloe vera cream

6 capsules vitamin E oil, or ½ teaspoon wheatgerm oil
4 teaspoons aloe vera gel
125 ml/4 fl oz/½ cup almond oil
1 tablespoon lanolin

Pierce capsules and add oil to the mixture of aloe vera gel and almond oil. Beat vigorously or use a blender to combine. Pour into a small bowl. Melt lanolin in a bain-marie (water bath) or a double saucepan (boiler). Take from the heat, add oil mixture and beat continuously until it is cool. Store in a glass jar.

Simple moisturizer

2 tablespoons almond oil
2 tablespoons rose-water

Mix the ingredients together vigorously. Shake well before use.

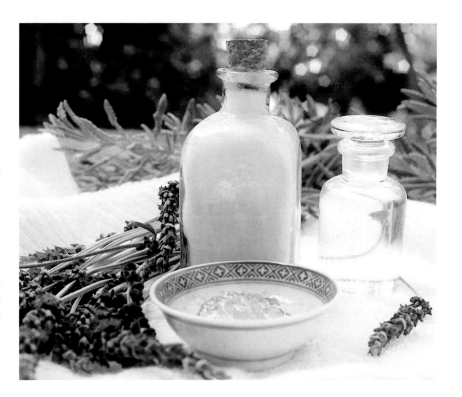

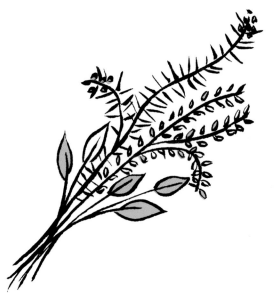

ABOVE:

Aloe vera gel is obtained from the succulent leaves of the aloe vera plant. It has marvellous healing properties and is used in many natural bodycare preparations.

OPPOSITE:

Always cleanse your face gently before applying moisturizers. Facial skin tissue is delicate and requires a soft, patting motion rather than energetic scrubbing.

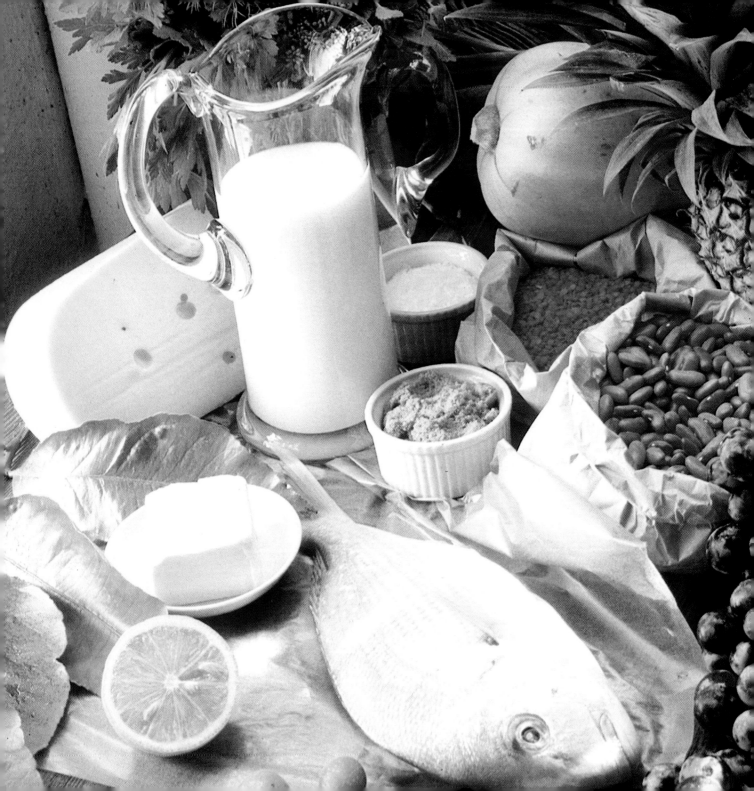

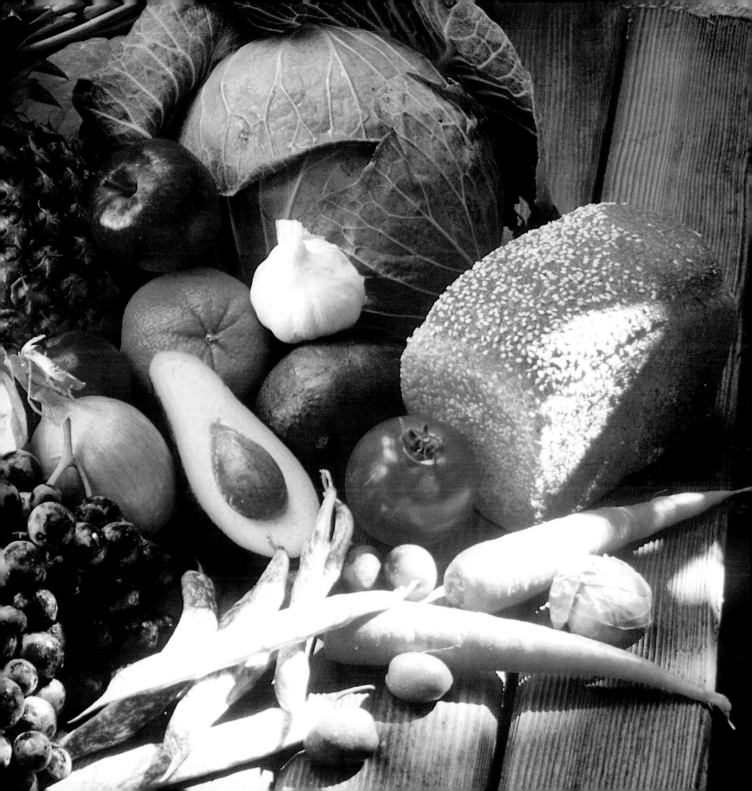

tip

Our skin ages naturally but of course we want to slow it down! The skin loses collagen, a protein from the dermis, and the fat below. The glands do not produce as much oil and moisture. Exercise, massage, cleansing, toning, moisturizers, sun protection, fluids and a highly nutritious diet all help the skin perform at its best – retaining vitality and glow for as long as humanly possible!

The body

Regular baths are probably the single best natural treatment you can give your skin – allowing sweat glands to release wastes, taking a load off the lymphatic system, softening dead cells for easy removal and relaxing all muscles, nerves and organs. Baths also prepare the skin for cleansers, toners or moisturizers. See page 14 for bath treatment techniques and ideas. Here are some extra tips.

Skin brushing

Before your bath or shower, try dry-skin body brushing – massage gently at first – to stimulate circulation and remove dead skin. Use a gentle downward movement for the first week or so to accustom skin to the procedure.

Simple additions to the bath

Aromatherapy oils can be used for many effects. For sheer pleasure, use rose, neroli and sandalwood; to stimulate circulation, rosemary and lemon; to soothe, pine, rose and camomile; and, as antiseptic agents, eucalyptus, tea-tree or thyme. Add only 5 to 10 drops. Herbal teas (see page 46) can also be added to the bath – 250 ml/8 fl oz/1 cup per bath.

You can add 1 teaspoon of different moisturizing oils to the water, such as almond or avocado, these can also be applied after a bath. Toning agents such as witch hazel or lemon juice will tighten the skin. Make up your own combinations or try the Herbal bath recipe opposite.

Moisturizers

Simple, cold-pressed oils or aloe vera gel can be used as a moisturizer. Our Simple moisturizer and Aloe vera cream (page 29) are great moisturizers. Avocado oil is a rich skin treatment before bedtime once a week. Shower off in the morning.

Recipes

Herbal bath

This combination of common herbs will give your skin a fresh look, toning the skin all over.

750 ml/1¼ pints/3 cups water
2 teaspoons dried mint
2 teaspoons rosemary
2 teaspoons sage
1 tablespoon lavender flowers
1 tablespoon witch hazel
1 tablespoon almond oil
Juice of ½ a fresh lemon

Bring the water to the boil and add all the dried herbs. Let them steep for 12 hours. Strain through muslin (cheesecloth) and add the witch hazel and almond oil. Discard the used herbs. Store in a tightly sealed glass container. Use 250 ml/8 fl oz/1 cup per bath. To finish, pour the lemon juice into the bath.

Aromatic water

Aromatic waters combine fragrant herbs with pure water and are used as body washes, skin toners and hair rinses. Use 3 drops of essential oil to 5 tablespoons water or try the recipe below.

12 drops jasmine
5 drops bergamot
3 drops lavender
600 ml/1 pint/2½ cups pure water

Always use distilled water, mineral water or rainwater. Add essential oils to water and mix well. Store in a glass container.

Mint water

This recipe has an alternative fragrance to rose-water on page 22.

6 tablespoons dried mint
600 ml/1 pint/2½ cups pure water

Crush mint and add to water in a glass jar with an airtight lid. Store conveniently so you can shake one to two times a day for two weeks. Strain and use.

Aromatic deodorant

Dilute essential oils with almond or wheatgerm oil to place on the body as a deodorant or perfume. Use 5 drops of essential oil to 125 ml/4 fl oz/½ cup of oil or water.

1 tablespoon rose-water
30 drops geranium
30 drops lavender
125 ml/4 fl oz/½ cup witch hazel
250 ml/8 fl oz/1 cup pure water

Mix all of the above ingredients thoroughly. Store in a glass container.

Witch hazel deodorant

½ teaspoon dried rosemary
½ teaspoon dried lavender
125 ml/4 fl oz/½ cup witch hazel

Steep herbs in witch hazel for 5 days then strain. If used as a hair rinse this can help in the treatment of dandruff.

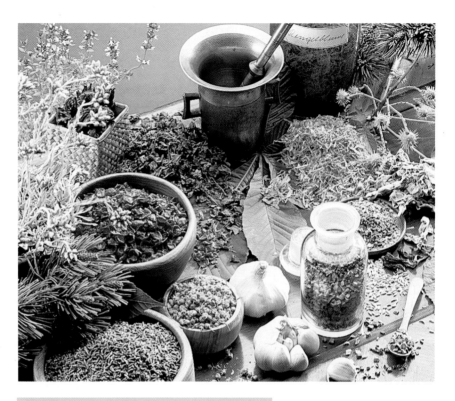

The hair

Hair is made of strong, elastic strands of the protein keratin. A special follicle just under the skin produces cells of keratin, which continuously divide and push up into the light. An oil gland lies beside the hair follicle, and lubricates both the hair and the skin.

There are approximately 100,000 hair follicles on the head and these produce hair in cycles. A follicle will be active for three to six years, shed the hair, rest, then begin to grow a new hair. We normally lose around 100 hairs from the head each day as old hairs make way for new. The hair cycle can be altered by major events such as surgery, childbirth, severe stress or chemotherapy. If diet and lifestyle are healthy it returns to normal after a few months.

Healthy hair needs good circulation and nutrient-rich blood. Adequate protein levels are important

ABOVE:
There is a wide variety of healing plants available. They come from trees, garden flowers, small shrubs and grasses, but they all share some common properties – plenty of vitamins and minerals, and the potential to provide aromatic essential oils.

tip

Natural henna for all hair types is an ancient conditioner! Slowly add 2 tablespoons of neutral henna to 600 ml/1 pint/2½ cups of cold water in a saucepan, mix continuously to form a cream. Heat gently for 3 minutes, stirring. Apply the warm mixture to your scalp, then work back through the hair. Cover with a plastic cap and leave for 1 hour. Rinse well!

as is a reasonable amount of vitamin A. Lack of the B vitamins during periods of stress can cause the hair to become dull, thin and dry.

Good hair hygiene will keep the scalp healthy and free from excessive build-up of oils. Brushing hair and massaging the scalp help – as does washing with a mild shampoo. Care for your scalp and hair ends separately. Too much exposure to wind and sun can damage hair, so wear a scarf or hat!

Dandruff treatments

Apple cider vinegar massaged into the scalp is an old-fashioned remedy for dandruff. Apply it warm, with cotton wool pads (swabs). Wrap your head in a towel for 30 minutes. Wash out the treatment with a shampoo. Or dilute the vinegar with water to make a rinse – 1 part vinegar to 6 parts water. Apply this solution morning and evening with a comb until the hair is soaked to assist an itching scalp.

A parsley infusion rubbed into the scalp helps shift dandruff if repeated. Vitamin E improves the health of scalp skin and B-complex vitamins fight dandruff. A highly nutritious diet is vital too.

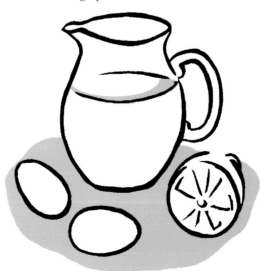

Recipes

Rosemary hair rinse

This rinse can add gloss to hair and reduce the build-up of static electricity. Replace the rosemary with nettle to ward off dandruff.

1 teaspoon dried (2 teaspoons fresh) rosemary
600 ml/1 pint/2½ cups boiling water

Add herbs to water and allow the infusion to steep for 15 minutes to 2 hours. Strain before using as a final rinse after shampoo.

As an additional rinse on an oily scalp try using 2 tablespoons lemon juice to 1 cup water. Massage this in well, then shampoo.

Old-fashioned shampoo

This is a very effective traditionally used recipe. As a variation, to combine as a conditioner, add 1 teaspoon of almond oil to the mixture and leave on the hair for at least 15 minutes before rinsing.

2 fresh eggs
1 teaspoon strained lemon juice
125 ml/4 fl oz/½ cup cool water
1 teaspoon almond oil, optional

All the ingredients should be at room temperature so that the eggs do not set. Blend together for one minute. Apply to wet hair, massaging well into the scalp for up to 10 minutes and spread the mixture thoroughly through your hair. Rinse well with cool water until all the egg has disappeared. Use a rosemary or lemon juice based rinse.

Aromatherapy for the scalp

This recipe stimulates the scalp and strengthens hair, reducing hair loss.

4 tablespoons almond oil
3 drops rosemary*
3 drops lavender*

Prepare and apply as in the preceding recipe, but leave in hair for 1 hour. Add shampoo to dry hair for better removal of oil. Replace aromatherapy oils* with juniper and cedarwood to assist with dandruff and oily hair.

Oil treatment for dry hair

This is an intensive treatment for dry hair using a blend of aromatherapy oils.

3 tablespoons almond oil (or other – wheatgerm, soya)
3 drops aromatherapy oil (camomile, rose)

Warm the oils gently and blend them together. Massage thoroughly into the scalp and spread throughout your hair, especially ensure that dried ends are covered. Cover the scalp with hot towels for 20 minutes. Rinse and shampoo thoroughly.

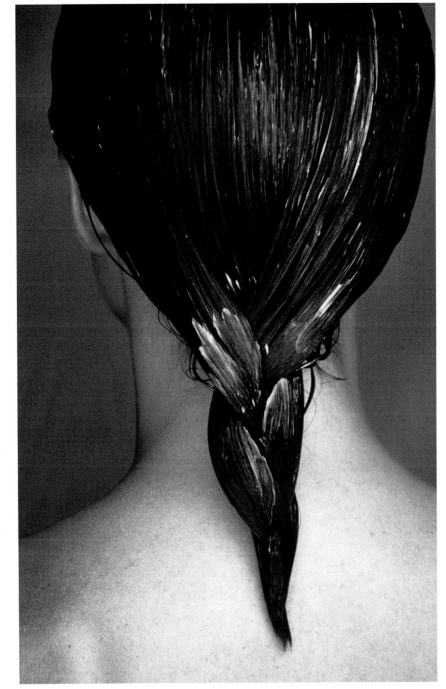

Body Preparations

*B*ody care is more than skin deep. Good posture, relaxed yet firm muscle tone and strong resilient nerves are all signs of a healthy body. Nervous and muscular tension can affect the health of the skin as well, altering blood supply and causing a greater demand on important nutrients.

Our chapter on Feeling Good, page 51, describes some simple exercise, massage, meditation and stress management techniques.

Nervous and muscular systems

There are some simple ways that you can use aromatic herbs to improve muscle tone and ease nervous tension.

First, baths and foot baths are highly recommended for improving, relaxing and toning our nervous and muscular systems. Consult the sections detailing the different kinds of bathing treatments you can use on pages 14 to 17. Follow up your bath with a soothing massage, trying out the following home-made oils.

Massage oils

In general, these are blends that aim to promote the circulation of blood and lymph, and improve skin health. You need a base oil in which to dissolve the aromatherapy oil.

The oil you choose must have the ability to penetrate into the skin, carrying the aromatic oil into the blood supply. Mineral oils such as baby oil do not penetrate very far, whereas a range of fine vegetable oils work very well. These must be 100 per cent pure, unrefined, cold-pressed oils, as good quality as you can afford. Vegetable oils usually contain vitamins A and E – excellent for the skin. All these features will ensure excellent penetration and a good shelf life.

Avocado oil is one of the best to choose and it can be diluted with other oils as it is fairly rich – good for dry skins. Olive, almond, soya, sunflower and grapeseed oils are all good base oils. Wheatgerm oil is expensive but very good at preserving the massage oil as it has vitamin E to inhibit the rancidity that tends to occur once the aromatic oils are added. Only make up 5 tablespoons at a time. Add 15 drops of the aromatic oil to the base oil. It is not good to either use too much, or to be too generous with essential oil. However, do not be afraid to experiment a little with the blend of oils to find the balance that you prefer.

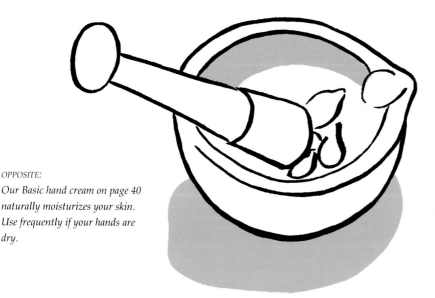

OPPOSITE:
Our Basic hand cream on page 40 naturally moisturizes your skin. Use frequently if your hands are dry.

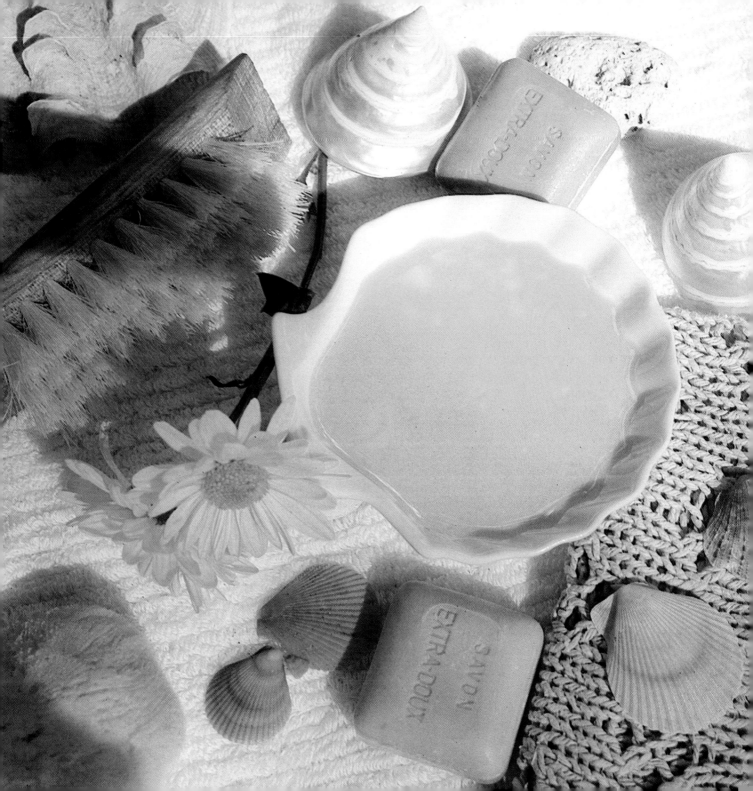

Recipes

Fragrant massage oil

The recipes below can be used to ease or relieve muscle tension and the associated mild aches. Although used for massage, all of these oils and combinations can be used in your bath – 5 to 10 drops per bath.

1 teaspoon avocado oil
1 teaspoon wheatgerm oil
5 tablespoons sunflower seed oil
5 drops lavender*
5 drops rosemary*
5 drops eucalyptus*

Use the basic recipe above and vary the ingredients for the following complaints:

NERVOUS TENSION – replace aromatic oils* with 5 drops each of lavender, sandalwood and orange blossom (neroli) oils, or with 5 drops each of cedar, sandalwood and bergamot oils.

RELAXING – replace aromatic oils* with 5 drops each of rose, camomile and geranium oils.

REFRESHING AND TONING – make a massage oil using 8 drops bergamot, with 4 drops each of jasmine and rose oils.

It is often good to experiment with one essential oil before mixing, so that you can establish its therapeutic benefits for yourself without confusion. Consult our Aromatherapy table and suggestions on page 21.

Hands and feet

The hands and feet probably suffer more from the rigours of daily life than other parts of the body.

The skin on the under surface of your hands and feet is quite different from the rest of your body – the epidermal layer is about ten times as thick as elsewhere and there is no hair. Because they are in so much contact with the environment, hands and feet need to be especially tough and resistant to injury and infection, as well as being very sensitive to many different stimuli. Consequently, they need a great deal of tender loving care, with hygiene being most important.

Hands and feet are made up of many fine bones and a complex sensory system of nerves, and an array of musculature for very delicate movement. Exercise and relaxation are also required, especially for the feet which bear your weight all day long.

Moisturizing

Use the Simple moisturizer (page 29) lavishly on hands and feet. Replace almond oil with glycerine for a more protective lotion. Lanolin is an old remedy to soften rough, chapped skin.

Diets rich in vitamins A, B complex and E also help the skin to replace itself as surface tissue becomes damaged, and helps to enhance the oil glands' ability to produce more oil. Extra oil in the diet may assist, but do not overdo it.

Protecting the hands

Always wear gloves with cotton lining when dish-washing or gardening and especially when exposed to any chemicals. Do not wear the gloves for more than 20 minutes at a time to avoid excessive perspiration.

Barrier cream is a useful protective substance. Apply hand cream or lotion regularly, at least four to six times a day. As an intensive night-time treatment, apply a heavy hand cream such as lanolin to your hands and wear cotton gloves. Wheatgerm, olive and vitamin E oil are also recommended, or try the recipe on the following page.

Nail care

Nails are tough protein shields, made from keratin, that protect the sensitive tips of your fingers and toes. They never stop growing and must be constantly trimmed.

Good nail nutrition involves many minerals in the diet – zinc, calcium, magnesium and iron, plus protein, vitamins A and B complex. Remember that nails grow very slowly so it will take at least four months to see the benefits.

Dry and brittle nails are often caused by too much contact with water. They do not have the ability to retain water that is temporarily absorbed, and consequently dry out. Therefore nails must be moisturized with creams and lotions.

Hang nails result from excessive dryness, injury or clumsy pushing back of the cuticle. Trim near the base of the hang nail and use an antiseptic oil such as tea-tree or thyme to inhibit infection. Apply the oil at least three times a day.

Foot bath treatments

To relax and soothe tired or sore feet, to stimulate circulation and decrease odour, try a foot bath using some of the following additives:

CEDAR OIL	to soothe feet
EPSOM SALTS	or a mixture of lavender and rosemary for tired aching feet
CIDER VINEGAR	1 part to 8 parts water as a regular treatment works well for foot odour
LAVENDER	suitable for perspiring feet

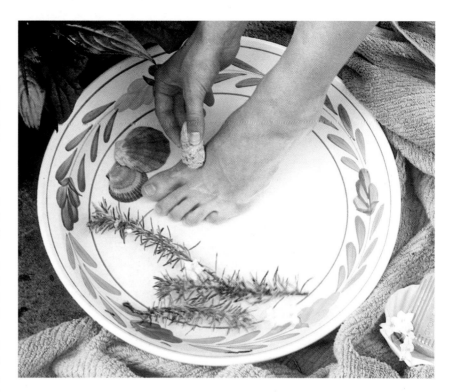

Start by soaking your feet for 15 minutes in a foot bath containing 5 to 10 drops of aromatherapy oil to 3 litres/5¼ pints/3½ quarts warm water.

Use pumice or a brush to loosen rough or dead skin from either your hands or feet after soaking them.

Massage the upper surface of the feet and knead underneath to release tension and aid circulation. Use almond or apricot kernel oil to massage your feet and lower legs, adding some essential oil as you wish. Try and experiment with reflexology see page 52.

Treat your toenails with the same care as your fingernails. Use a soothing moisturizer on the nails. Trim nails straight and file edges. Ingrown toenails usually result from either cutting the nails too close or wearing tight shoes. If a nail becomes infected, see your doctor.

ABOVE:
Ease tired and aching feet with warm, fragrant foot baths while you read or watch television. Foot baths are also good for headaches.

Recipes

Basic hand cream

Experiment with lanolin quantities for desired strength. Camomile or rose oil are soothing.

2 tablespoons lanolin
2 tablespoons almond or wheatgerm oil
4 drops soothing essential oil of your choice

Heat lanolin gently in a double saucepan (boiler), stirring well. When liquid, remove from heat and add almond oil and essential oil, stirring until cool. Store in a glass jar.

Weekly fingernail treat

Place fingers in a solution of lemon juice and warm water for 5 minutes. If they are very dry, place in warm olive, almond or wheatgerm oil for 10 to 15 minutes.

Towel dry and rub a lotion or cream into each nail with a circular motion to encourage circulation and soften the cuticle so it can be gently eased back. Always rub extra lotion into your cuticles and treat them very gently. Lanolin is also good for brittle nails.

The mouth

It is tremendously important to maintain adequate hygiene in your mouth – for good digestion as well as pleasant breath. Healthy teeth and gums rely on healthy mouth tissue, full of nutrient-rich blood and free from as many harmful bacteria as possible.

B-complex vitamins and vitamin C are important to the mouth. Boost foods containing these vitamins in your diet if you have any mouth soreness. Various mouth washes and gargles assist by keeping the chemistry of the mouth balanced. Yoghurts supplying friendly bacteria keep the mouth in good health. The health of the mouth, especially that of the tongue, often reflects the health of the whole digestive system. Yoghurt also alleviates bad breath. In addition, we need to use antiseptic mouthwashes to destroy harmful bacteria.

1

tip

Ancient remedies to sweeten the breath include sucking whole cloves, chewing anise seed, cardamom or a piece of nutmeg! Or just eat a leaf or two from your mint plant in passing! Parsley is also good, as are fenugreek and peppermint tea.

Mouthwashes and gargles

These are useful in staving off infections. Tea-tree oil in warm water makes an excellent gargle because it is such a good antibiotic. Salt-water gargles are also effective. Sage oil and warm sage infusion are recommended as a soothing gargle, sage being a mild antiseptic. A mixture of lemon, myrrh and sage oil makes a good all-purpose mouthwash or gargle. Use 3 to 6 drops essential oil in 1 cup warm water to make up your mouthwash.

Teeth care

The obvious opportunity to improve oral hygiene is when you clean your teeth. Taking good care of teeth and gums will benefit the rest of the mouth. Healthy teeth need healthy gums above all. The most important factor is not when you brush your teeth, but how you brush your teeth.

The gums need to be brushed as well as the tongue! It may seem a little strange to you if you have not tried this. Yet this is the very best way of stimulating circulation and cleaning away the thick layers of plaque (invisible sticky deposits of bacteria) coating the gums and tongue.

If plaque is removed effectively at least once a day, it does not get the opportunity to do a great deal of damage. See the illustrations below on good brushing technique.

Calcium and other minerals including magnesium and zinc, help to promote healthy teeth by working from the inside out. Vitamin C aids the fight against bacteria. Eating raw vegetables is an excellent way to exercise teeth and gums, as well as provide valuable nutrients.

Clove oil applied directly to the gum gives an effective, if temporary, relief from toothache.

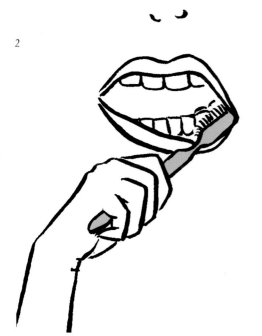

2

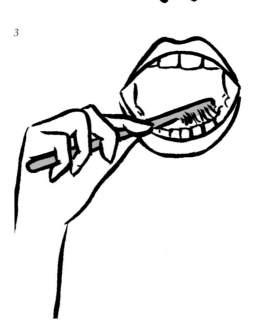

3

GUMLINE BRUSHING TECHNIQUE: Always use soft toothbrushes for this gumline brushing technique. Floss gently too. A little bleeding may occur the first few times you use these techniques – if it continues, check with your dentist.

1 *Floss teeth regularly.*
2 *Place the brush firmly along the line where teeth meet gums. Wriggle the brush back and forth with short movements. The tips will penetrate into the gaps between the teeth and along the gum line.*
3 *Roll brush down teeth to remove remaining plaque. For molars, press firmly down and vibrate.*

OPPOSITE:
Tired eyes need special treatment. Eye balms and compresses soothe tired skin and muscles. A slice of cucumber placed over each eye is a simple and effective eye balm. If skin is sensitive, protect with a light oil.

tip

Simple ways to relieve eye strain include covering the eyes gently with your fingers to create darkness. Do not push! Slowly move your eyes from left to right, up, down; rotate, raising and lowering eyebrows! Improve your focusing by concentrating on your hand at 10 cm/4 inches, then at a distant horizon. Gently repeat. Always move your eyes as much as possible when driving long distances.

The nose, ears and eyes

The nose

Blocked noses benefit tremendously from inhalations. Eucalyptus oil alone or mixtures that contain it are best. These are known as decongestants, stimulating the body to clear mucus, which usually forms as a result of extra bacterial activity. It is also possible to rinse the nasal passages, usually with salty water, but most people find the sensation a little unusual.

The ears

The ears are delicate instruments and need special care. First, protect your ears from specially loud noises. Second, keep a check on the build-up of ear wax, whose job is to trap bacteria, dirt and dust and lubricate the ear canal. Warm almond oil can soften ear wax and it will fall out of its own accord. Sometimes you may need to get your ears syringed by the doctor. Warm almond oil will soothe earache. Use a dropper – 2 drops in each ear.

For lightly blocked ears, use either of the following. Place a finger at the front of the ear and firmly massage the closed ear canal. Alternatively, lightly pinch the nose, close the mouth, then try to blow your nose. A faint click indicates that your ears have acclimatized to the pressure change.

The eyes

Vitamin A, lemon grass tea and carrot juice are good for the eyes. The B-complex vitamins and vitamins C and E are needed for eye care. Delicate oils full of vitamin E are good for the eye area. Apply carefully and regularly for the best effect. Try the following herbal remedies to soothe tired eyes. These aim to soothe eye muscles and rejuvenate delicate skin. Keep fluid out of the eye. At the slightest sign of irritation cease treatment.

Recipes

Compresses

Use potato for circles and bags, and apple for tired eyes. Grate raw, and place it in moist muslin (cheesecloth). Place over eyes for 15 minutes. Always make up fresh.

Eye balms

Cotton wool pads (swabs) dipped in cool water, milk or a herbal infusion are simple to apply. Try using parsley, fennel or camomile. Make up the infusion as on page 22.

Puffy eyes will benefit from (cool) camomile tea bags! An old favourite is to place a slice of cucumber over each eye. Lie down and give yourself at least 15 minutes to absorb the full benefits.

Inhalations

5 drops eucalyptus*
3 drops peppermint*
2 drops sage or thyme*
½ bowl boiling water

Prepare and apply as described in the Water therapy section (pages 14 and 16). This recipe is a very good decongestant. For a general antiseptic, and to cleanse bronchial passages, replace the above essential oils* with 5 drops eucalyptus and 3 drops each lavender and sandalwood oils.

Other antiseptic oils described on page 21 will also work well. Spicy food can also work as a decongestant.

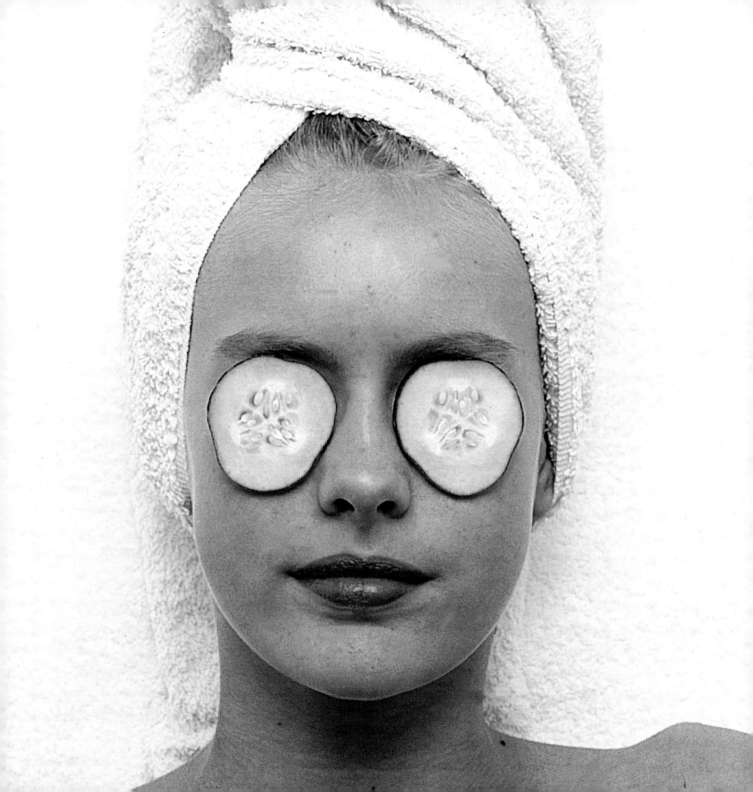

Natural Health Care

*V*arious herbs, aromatic oils and health foods can be used in the home to relieve minor complaints.

Subtle changes in the body indicate that some deterioration is beginning to occur. If you know

how to respond quickly, you may prevent a more serious condition developing. Most natural therapies

rely on teaching people to prevent illness and become more observant of their bodily functions.

Small, everyday actions can make a considerable difference to your health. Natural remedies are

often used in conjunction with normal medical procedures. For example, if you are taking antibiotics,

make sure you follow up afterwards with yoghurt to build up your own supply of healthy bacteria again.

D o not delay seeking professional health advice if you suspect the development of a problem.

There is increasing co-operation developing between the medical profession and alternative health practitioners. After all, many modern drugs come from plants and herbs. As a patient, always ensure that all of the avenues available to you are explored thoroughly.

Do not hesitate to discuss natural health care with your doctor and, similarly, do justice to benefits you receive from modern medical discoveries when

consulting natural health professionals. In this way we can work toward a time when we will all automatically have access to the best of both worlds.

We have been careful to describe only the most common and widely recognized natural health care products and remedies. If you have not tried these remedies before, begin with one substance at a time, monitoring yourself as you go. There is such a vast range of herbs in the world and so many different supplements and new discoveries appearing on the market, it can be rather confusing to begin with.

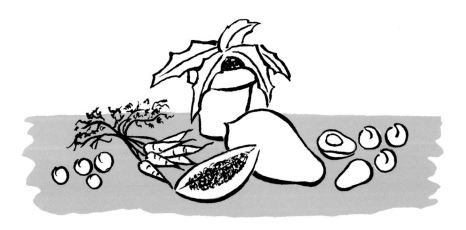

OPPOSITE:

Herbal teas are not only medicinal. They are delicious hot or cold and can even be drunk with milk. Always follow preparation instructions for the best results.

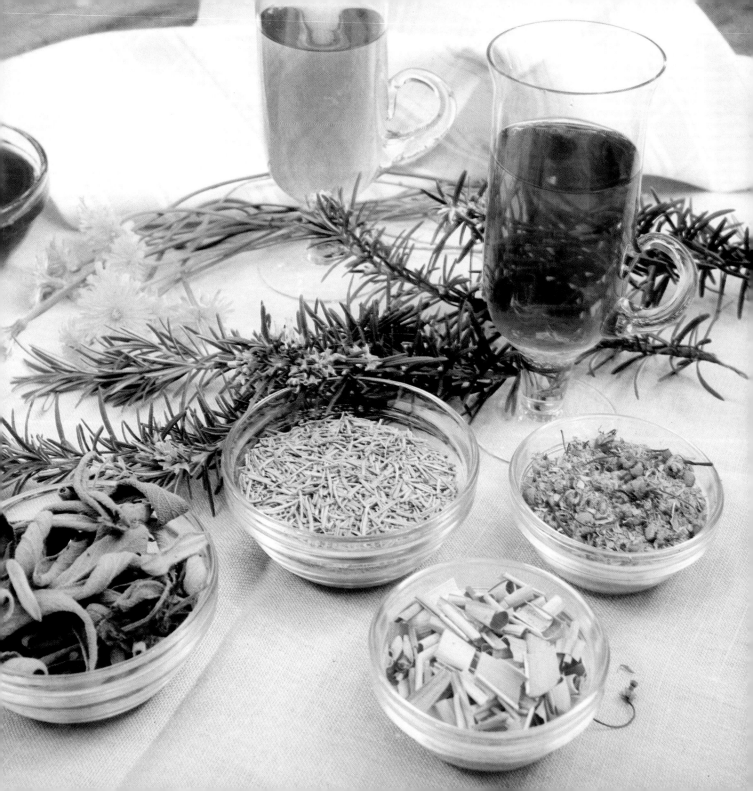

Herbal teas

CAMOMILE
A mild, delightful tea (do not brew too long); calms nerves and aids the mucus lining of all inner systems, good for easing menstrual pain.

DANDELION
A very pleasant hot drink, substitute for coffee; said to stimulate liver function and eliminate wastes; aids digestion.

LEMON GRASS
A hot or cold drink as a tonic for the kidneys and skin; contains vitamin A.

PEPPERMINT
A stimulating drink; taken after meals, it assists digestion; relieves gas; good for coughs and colds.

RASPBERRY LEAF
A mild tea; remedy for minor problems in pregnant women and new mothers; relieves nausea.

ROSEHIP
A tangy drink; high in vitamin C which assists lymphatic system fight germs; relieves skin infections.

ROSEMARY
A fragrant tea; used as a stomach and nerve tonic; aids memory.

SAGE
A savoury tea; assists brain, nerve and liver function; said to aid concentration.

Common health foods and products

ALFALFA SPROUTS
Rich in calcium, phosphorus, magnesium, potassium, and vitamins A, B complex, C, D and E. Eat for nervous or digestive disorders.

ALOE VERA
A wonderful fast skin healer; remedy for sunburn, cuts, burns, rashes, insect bites, blisters and body odour; great for healthy skin too.

APRICOT KERNEL OIL
Rich in copper and unsaturated fats; excellent tonic for the blood and for dry skin; use in salads or massage oils. Do not heat.

AVOCADO OIL
Contains vitamins A, B complex and C, iron and potassium; excellent penetration of skin, offering good protection against wind and sun; excellent base for massage oil.

BREWERS' YEAST
An excellent source of B-complex vitamins, other vitamins and minerals; excellent tonic; good for stress, nervous complaints, skin irritation and tired eyes. Avoid if you have candida.

CARROT JUICE
Contains a full range of minerals and beta carotene (for vitamin A); excellent for healing skin; tonic during stress; said to relieve arthritis.

EUCALYPTUS OIL
A decongestant which helps to relieve a blocked nose and blocked sinuses, colds and congested chests; use as mouthwash, for muscular pain and insect bites; generally stimulates circulation.

tip

Aloe vera is a cactus that has a marvellous soothing gel inside its leaves – a great instant remedy for many minor skin problems such as insect bites, rashes, swellings, burns, cuts, scratches and sunburn. Take large base leaves and cut/peel away rind to reveal gel. Apply gel directly to a cleaned wound to provide a protective covering that assists healing. Also available in health food shops.

EVENING PRIMROSE OIL
Rich in a fatty acid usually only found in human milk; maintains circulation and healthy arteries; good for skin complaints and premenstrual tension (PMT).

GARLIC
A natural antibiotic, said to treat infections and remove toxins from the blood; stimulates digestion; contains vitamins A, B complex and C, copper, calcium and iron.

GINSENG
A general tonic, said to strengthen heart and nervous system, increasing vitality and resistance to disease.

KELP
Is used to improve hormonal balance, as it contains so many minerals, especially iron and iodine, and vitamins A, B complex and E.

LAVENDER OIL
Soothes muscles and nerves, can reduce effect of burns, but not pain; effective pimple treatment, apply directly to pimples.

LECITHIN
Aids digestion; nourishes nerves; assists vitamins A and E uptake; may prevent cholesterol build-up; high in phosphorus.

PAPAYA (PAWPAW) OINTMENT
Rich in many vitamins and minerals; soothes and heals cuts, open sores, bruises, cracked skin on lips and feet, and detergent allergies.

TEA-TREE OIL
A natural antibiotic; use in inhalations to help prevent skin infections; effective pimple treatment, apply 2–3 times daily.

TIGER BALM
An almost instant relief for muscular and nerve pain, and headaches; apply tiny amounts to pressure points; avoid sensitive skin areas.

TOFU
A soya bean curd containing low-fat protein; easily digestible; its bland flavour allows it to be used in both savoury and sweet dishes.

VALERIAN
A wonderful remedy for calming the nervous system; especially good for insomnia and stomach cramp; comes in tablets or tea.

WHEATGERM
High in protein, vitamin B complex and E, iron, phosphorus and other minerals; a great general tonic for the skin; wheatgerm oil is the highest known source of vitamin E.

WITCH HAZEL
An antiseptic and skin toner; provides temporary relief from varicose veins and pressure in legs; use double distilled.

YOGHURT
Yoghurt is made from milk cultured with bacteria naturally present in the intestines; it is high in protein, vitamins A, B complex and D; replaces friendly bacteria after digestive problems or use of antibiotics; largely lactose-free; use in sweet and savoury dishes and drinks.

tip

Women who suffer from premenstrual tension (PMT) and pain can benefit from natural remedies. Camomile tea, evening primrose oil, kelp, yeast and food sources of vitamin B6, wholegrain cereals, fresh vegetables, bananas and cabbage will assist you! You are aiming to alter the whole way your body responds to this natural change in rhythm so there is a smooth transition! Meditation and gentle exercise also help relax you emotionally and physically.

Key vitamins and minerals

Vitamin and mineral supplements help to make up for inadequacies in the diet. Often people take supplements when they are unwell. Food is the best source of these nutrients, because the body is designed to digest and absorb the vitamins and minerals naturally from fresh fruit and vegetables, and whole grains.

Many vitamins are water-soluble and easily lost during soaking or cooking. These are an important part of your diet and need to be constantly replaced. They include the B-group vitamins and vitamin C. Vitamins A, D and E are fat-soluble and need some fat to be digested effectively. Vitamin C, vitamin B12 and folic acid are very sensitive to air, light and heat. Always make sure that you prepare and store food containing these vitamins carefully. Vitamin C and vitamin E are notable antioxidants, protecting your system from toxic substances.

Following is a list of the major vitamins and minerals and what they do for your body.

Vitamins and minerals table

B-COMPLEX VITAMINS

They often work together and occur together in food. Essential for metabolism of fat, protein and carbohydrate; vital for energy and for the health of the nervous system and brain.

B1 THIAMINE

Converts glucose to energy; assists heart, brain and nerve function; thought to improve learning capacity.

B2 RIBOFLAVIN

Helps digestion; essential for good vision, skin, nails and hair.

B3 NIACIN

Used in the production of energy; important to nerve and brain function, blood, and digestive systems.

B12 & FOLIC ACID

Used in the production of blood, energy and cells; used by immune and nervous systems.

VITAMIN A

Aids growth and repair of body tissue (skin, inner mucous linings); fights disease and effects of pollutants; maintains eye health.

VITAMIN C

Strengthens tissue in skin, ligaments and joints; fights bacterial and viral infections; heals wounds; relieves allergy problems.

VITAMIN D

Involved in bone and tooth formation; stabilizes the nervous system; aids heart and blood action.

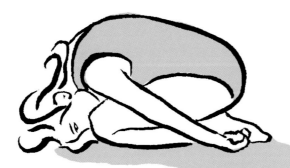

YOGA CHILD'S POSE FOR PMT:
This yoga position, known as the child's pose, relieves pre-menstrual tension. Stretch your spine, close your eyes and hold as long as is comfortable.

VITAMIN E
Prevents the breakdown of important nutrients; vital in the healing of skin, hormone production, and muscle and nerve function.

CALCIUM
Builds bones and teeth; aids nerve and muscle function, and the heartbeat; relieves insomnia.

COPPER
Important for blood formation and skin repair; is an antioxidant.

IODINE
Aids metabolism; involved in brain development; used by the thyroid gland.

IRON
An essential part of the haemoglobin that carries oxygen in the blood; improves muscle operation and the immune system; reduces stress.

MAGNESIUM
Aids the work of vitamin C and minerals; used as a muscle relaxant.

PHOSPHORUS
Essential for all processes; aids brain function; is involved in the formation of teeth and bones.

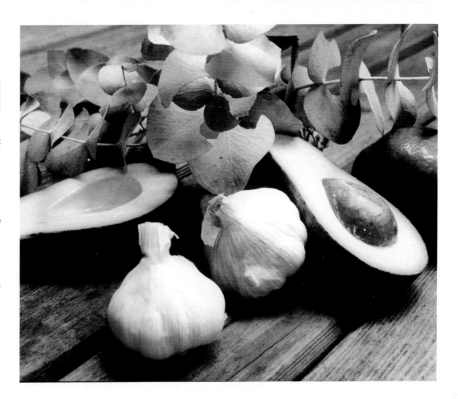

POTASSIUM
Helps regulate the body's water balance; assists nerve and muscle function.

SODIUM
Helps regulate the body's water balance; important to blood, nervous, muscle and lymph systems.

ZINC
Essential to most processes, especially reproduction, wound-healing and brain function.

ABOVE:
Both avocado and garlic are rich in vitamins and minerals and are good for your skin.

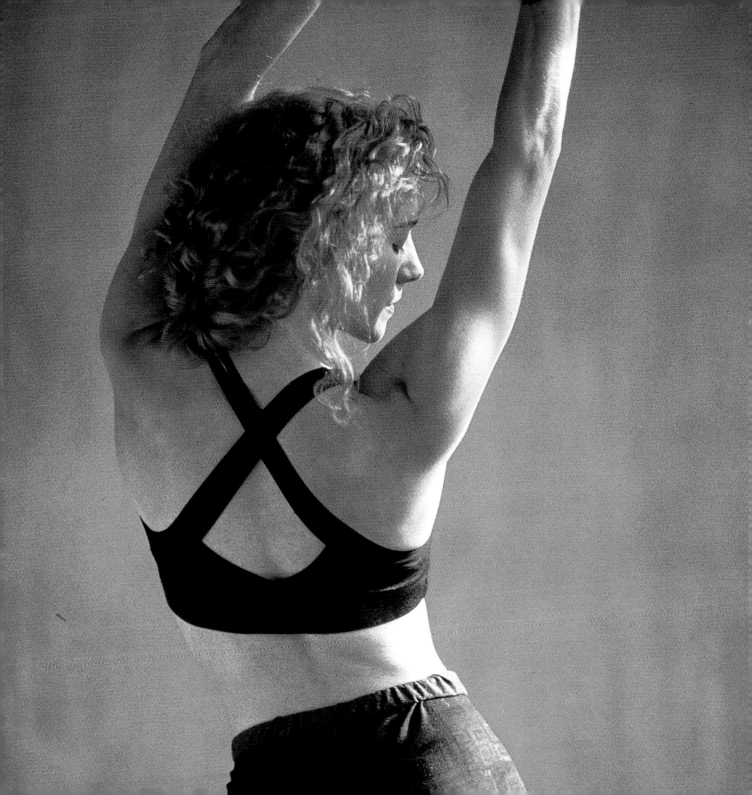

Feeling Good

*O*n the one hand we are what we eat. The content and the range of products that we consume affect our inner health and thus our outer being. It is the careful selection and monitoring of these elements that forms a solid base for how we feel about ourselves.

There are other important aspects of body care. Eating well on its own is not enough. To help you look your best and feel wonderful about yourself, you need to give some thought to keeping active, to relaxation and to establishing a positive outlook.

Exercise and massage

Exercise and massage are wonderful ways to stimulate the body's natural hygiene system to process and release its wastes. The lymphatic system relies on muscular movement to pump the fluid along. The skin's sweat glands perspire wastes and must constantly process fluids to maintain a healthy skin condition. Prolonged inactivity can result in blockages and infections of the cleansing systems.

The blood too will supply fresh nutrients to all parts of the body, as energetic aerobic exercise increases oxygen delivered to all cells. Office work uses certain muscles repeatedly, but leaves others without exercise. Stress and environmental pollution create other burdens.

Exercise and massage even out the use of muscles in the body, resulting in a well-toned, balanced feeling. Begin gradually if you have not done much exercise or massage recently.

Aerobic exercise

Aerobic exercise involves a steady but marked increase in the breathing rate, hence oxygen consumption, blood flow, muscle movement, perspiration and organ stimulation. It also improves strength and stamina. You need strong muscles to support your body, otherwise joints are placed under too much strain.

STAMINA – is staying power over a period of time and depends on strong lungs and heart. Regular aerobic exercise at least three to five times a week maintains a good fitness level.

WALKING – is an effective form of aerobic exercise, almost as effective as jogging, providing you walk regularly at a good pace to extend yourself. Thirty minutes five times a week will provide health benefits such as strengthening the heart, reducing blood pressure and increasing lung capacity.

Walking is so easy and requires only a good pair of shoes. You can pace yourself too, pausing now and then to stretch. Walking can be a time of reflection, a chance to gossip with a friend or an opportunity not to use the car every day.

SWIMMING – is an easy exercise involving very little equipment. A good pair of goggles is necessary in chlorinated pools. The water holds you up as you swim and has a unique total toning effect on all muscles of the body. As an exercise swimming is relaxing, invigorating and assists cleansing.

Moving evenly through the water increases stamina and strength without strain. The rhythmic

OPPOSITE:
Limber up with stretch exercises before intensive physical activity. Pace yourself during exercise by pausing to do stretches.

REFLEXOLOGY MAP:
When the soles of the feet are
massaged, reflex reactions are
triggered in different parts of the
body. Use this chart as a guide.

1   *Sinus*
2   *Pituitary gland*
3   *Stomach*
4   *Lungs*
5   *Kidneys*
6   *Pancreas*
7   *Spine*
8   *Large intestine*

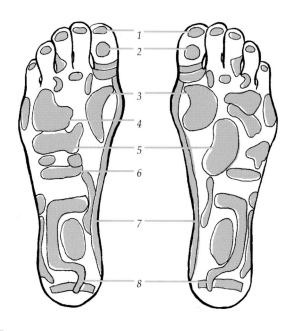

tip

Beauty without cruelty – opposition to product testing on animals is steadily rising. In fact many ingredients have already been tested before, and do not require retesting. Other forms of testing can be developed. Make your own products at home or vote with your money in this debate! We can only convince big business and government to alter their ethical standards by altering ours.

action of the water against your body stimulates circulation and conditions the muscles. Remember to vary your strokes to condition different muscles or try doing exercises in the water or underwater acrobatics! A good goal to aim for is 20 to 30-minute sessions, three to five times a week.

MOTIVATION – is not hard to come by when you choose a form of exercise you actually enjoy. Aim to achieve sensible rather than dramatic improvements in your fitness level, with the emphasis on reward rather than punishment!

Develop an interest that needs plenty of energetic movement – gardening, tennis, dancing, cycling, hiking, golf or wind surfing. Fun exercise that is available in gyms includes squash, aerobics, weight training or martial arts. Ideally, you should aim to exercise aerobically every day to maintain fitness and enthusiasm.

Stretching

Stretching is good for your health. Try to stretch on a regular basis to increase your flexibility. Muscles will remain elastic and joints move easily through their full range. You obtain better balance and posture, which contributes to how good you feel. Five to 10 minutes of stretch exercises a day increases energy and endurance, relieves many aches and pains and prevents long-term health problems.

You can easily fit stretch exercises into your daily routine. Start the day by limbering up with stretches that extend your arms and legs. This prepares your body for movement. There is usually more time in the evenings for floor exercises and yoga which strengthen your hips and back.

Massage

Massage has been practised through the ages to maintain the body's symmetry and equilibrium. Many different approaches are available from professional masseurs, courses and books. It is easy to experiment with simple massage techniques – begin working on yourself or with a friend, using our home-made massage oil on page 38.

REFLEXOLOGY – is a delightful, rather unusual form of foot massage that works on the Chinese principle that a complex nadi system, or energy network, lies adjacent to the nervous system and connects different parts of the body. In reflexology, special points on the soles of the feet are massaged in order to trigger a reflex action in those areas of the system to which they are connected. The chart shows the sensitive areas on the feet and names some of the organs believed to be linked with them.

The feet are very sensitive and can become overtired. In fact, any type of foot massage will soothe your feet and relax you all over. A foot massage is especially relaxing after a foot bath (see page 16).

SHIATSU – is an Eastern massage technique that works on the whole body. The massage follows the energy or nadi lines linking the different parts of the body as explained for reflexology.

First, soft, flowing effleurage is used, stroking the body with the whole hand, always making deeper strokes towards the heart to improve the flow of blood. Kneading follows – that is, pressure with the fingertips on tender spots where the nadi system is thought to be blocked. Shiatsu is also known as acupressure and is related to Chinese acupuncture, a system that uses tiny needles to relieve blockages at pressure points in the energy system.

SELF MASSAGE – is for the relief of tension and muscle strain. The neck and shoulder area often becomes quite sore and tight after desk work or lifting. If possible, loosen your muscles in a shower or bath first. You can massage the head and neck area quite effectively under the shower. Massage can also relieve headaches – try using the acupressure points illustrated below.

Meditation and stress management

Learning to relax consciously amidst the hustle and bustle of city life is quite an art. Yet many people are realizing that this is what they need to do to preserve the extra buoyancy and good spirits that make all the difference during rough times.

Restless nights, too much smoking and drinking, not having time to eat and digest good food, excessive worry and nervous tension – all of these stress symptoms can be alleviated if you take regular opportunities to relax and recuperate. They need only be brief moments, but they can be crucial to your long-term well-being.

Biologically, our bodies need adequate rest and periods of peace to allow healing and cleansing to occur, free from the strains of movement, digestion and dealing with other people. Our bodies need rest for nourishing tired muscles and repairing tissues, carrying away toxins and wastes and fighting off harmful micro-organisms.

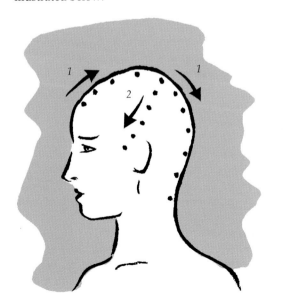
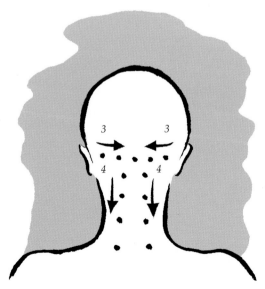

HEAD MASSAGE:
You can relieve a headache by pressing the points on line 1, along the middle of your head, followed by those along line 2 to the temples, doing both sides simultaneously. Follow with lines 3 and 4 down to the neck area.

You can aid this process by learning to relax from time to time during the day so that tension does not build up too high.

Baths which include aromatherapy oils also help. Soothing herbal teas will aid digestion and calm nerves. B-complex vitamins are the vitamins best suited to ease nervous symptoms. A highly nutritious diet replaces all the energy, minerals and vitamins that the body devours under stress.

Try to make time during the day to relieve nervous and emotional stress. Not only will you feel better but also you will find that you are able to counteract some of the immediate stress at work and at home.

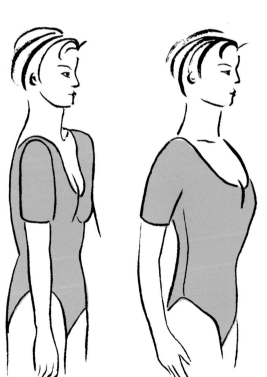

*SHOULDER SHRUGS FOR TENSION:
The head is quite heavy so the neck and shoulder area rapidly accumulates tension! Always stretch this area and massage it well under the shower.*

At work

Every so often, perform simple stretches to relieve muscle tension, or take a brief stroll. You can even lie down on the floor briefly, shoes off and feet slightly raised to refresh.

Have your lunch in a different place, a nearby park or sunny spot. Pace yourself to get in to work a little early or leave time for a visit to the local pool. Many people find exercise a wonderful way to relieve tension. Use a little incense or an ionizer to offset air conditioning. Place touches of beauty around you – a postcard, pot plant or humorous notes and wise sayings! There is more to life than work and you need time to relax

At home

Massage with deliciously fragrant oils is very soothing and relaxing. Regular, long, warm baths have the same effect. Walking, reading books, listening to music, exercise, gentle stretches in the mornings and evenings – all can change the pace of your life, giving the body a chance to rebalance. Brief naps and plenty of sleep help. Wearing vivid or mellow colours, depending on your mood, can also help to keep you balanced.

Try to put some special time aside to relax and refocus yourself by practising meditation, or perhaps one of the more reflective eastern arts like yoga or t'ai chi.

Simple relaxing meditation

In essence, meditation is a form of mental and emotional training. You allow yourself to discard old and unwanted thought patterns and relax any emotional turmoil. Be patient as you learn this art as it does take a little while to truly experience the benefits. Once you meditate regularly, however – even five to ten minutes a day – it gets easier and becomes a source of creative strength.

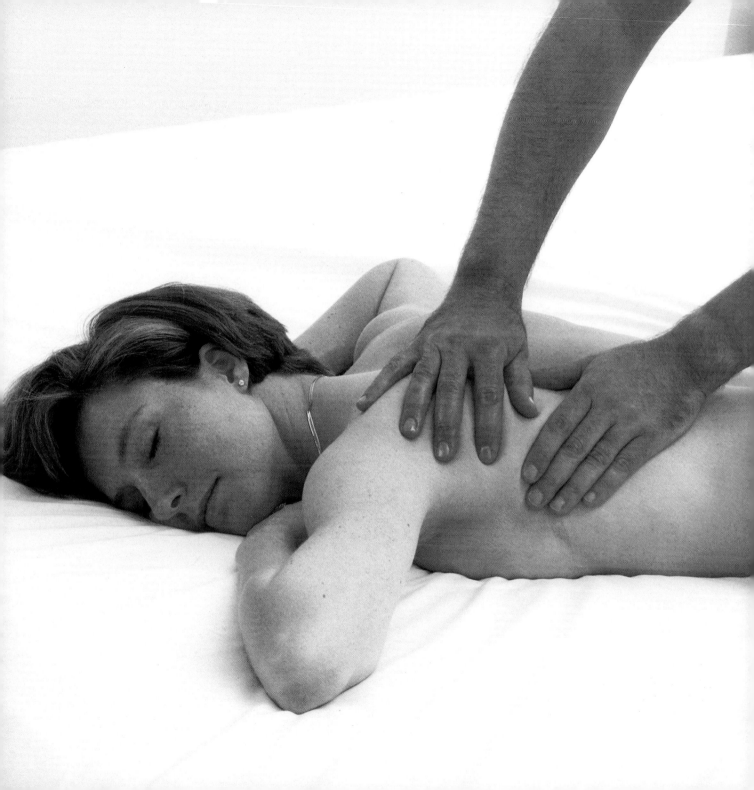

OPPOSITE:
Meditation relaxes the body and emotions, and clears the mind. A peaceful environment allows you to reach and maintain a peaceful meditative state.

Meditation can provide fresh ideas, breakthroughs for difficult personal problems and practical solutions to daily challenges at work. It is also an opportunity for your body to relax completely and refresh itself.

Start by wearing loose clothing and finding a quiet, comfortable place to sit where your spine is straight. You can use cushions on the floor and rest against the wall, or find a chair with good support. Sit in the same place each time while you are learning. Light some incense to inspire and relax you, if you like. It is a good idea to meditate at the same time each day, when you know you can avoid interruptions. Relaxing music may help you slow down before you begin.

You can plan ahead. The idea is to focus on a positive image or idea and actively imagine yourself experiencing it. It can be a simple saying, such as 'I am calm and content', or the mental picture of a beautiful country scene where you are sitting at peace – a forest, perhaps, where you can see the trees and flowers, feel the sun and hear the birds call.

It is best to sit still and begin to relax your body. Close your eyes and take a few deep breaths. Sometimes systematically tensing, then relaxing, each section of the body, from toes to head, helps to ease muscle tension – but do not spend too long doing this. Instead, picture showers of refreshing, clear light, cleansing you from head to toe, washing away all the tension and all the habitual negative thoughts. Let clear white, electric blue or gold coloured light flood through and around you for a few minutes. If you have trouble visualizing these colours, you can look out for them during the day and 'save them up' for your time of meditation.

After a few minutes, begin concentrating on the idea or image you have selected, picturing yourself in a peaceful location (with all the details) or imagining yourself calm and content. Often, other thoughts and feelings can intrude – simply acknowledge them and let them go. It can be a little disheartening at first if they disturb your concentration, but do not fight them – simply accept them, and they will gradually pass away. Concentrating for five minutes is enough at the beginning. As you practise each day, you become better at reaching a more peaceful meditative state and can maintain it for longer. Aim for 10 to 20 minutes each day. This can give you a clearer, more creative mind, a better perspective and even more relaxed breathing.

Other meditative approaches

Classes can teach you other basic styles. Zen meditation emphasizes breathing, whereas Transcendental Meditation focuses on a mantra, a simple word you repeat to quieten your mind. Listening to tape recordings of calming sounds is another popular method.

Gardening, praying, painting, playing music and other creative activities also stimulate the meditative faculties of the mind.

YOGA CORPSE POSITION:
The yoga corpse pose is deeply relaxing. Palms should be upturned and heels slightly apart. Breathe slowly and deeply, releasing all tensions.

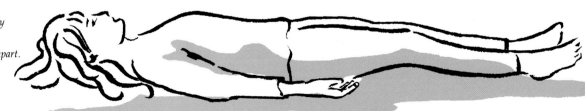

Eating well

A well-balanced, highly nutritious diet is essential for a healthy body. You need carbohydrates and protein for energy and building tissues. Constant supplies of vitamins and minerals are vital for all chemical processes. The right kinds of foods boost the body's immune and cleansing processes, some being particularly good for the skin. Healthy eating is needed in our modern life with its increased pace. Awareness of food and its particular role can remedy some health problems before they become serious.

Natural and fresh

Fresh and natural food is generally far better for us. Fresh fruit and vegetables are high-quality sources of important vitamins – many break down if heated, exposed to light or stored too long. There is far more food value in a whole apple than one cut up and cooked.

Our digestion works better if the muscles have fibre to push against – highly processed foods like white flour, rice or sugar, while rapidly digested, often do not go hand in hand with healthy bowels. Foods high in fibre include fresh fruit and vegetables, all grains and cereals such as brown bread, rice, oats and the pulses. Soluble fibre can help reduce cholesterol levels.

This does not mean we have to eat everything raw! But it is essential to balance cooked dishes with fresh fruit and salads – particularly in winter when less fresh produce is available, and there is less inclination to eat cold foods. However, with a little creativity they can be combined with tasty meals. Chopped parsley is a good source of vitamin C and can be added to many savoury dishes. Juiced vegetables and fruits are high in vitamins and minerals, a big boost for the immune system which generally works overtime in the colder months.

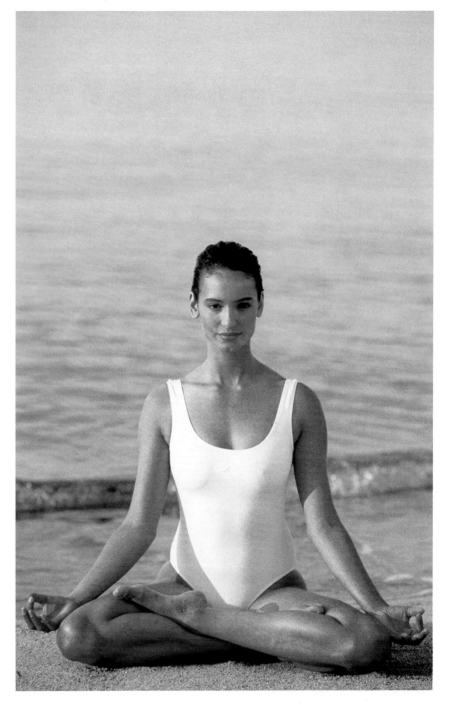

Balance

We need to eat the correct proportion of foods for a healthy diet, neither too much nor too little. This makes it far easier for the body to do its work – providing energy, building new cells to replace the old ones, cleansing itself and fighting disease. If too much of one food group is eaten, system overload occurs; too little and the body may not be able to make an important molecule. To make haemoglobin, for example, we must eat iron.

Eat some food every day from each of the five food groups to cover your body's basic needs.

Breads and cereals (group 1) and *fruits and vegetables* (group 2) should be eaten most often. Eat *meat and meat alternatives* (group 3) and *dairy products* (group 4) only moderately. *Oils and fats* (group 5), *sugar and salt* are required least of all.

Always vary your food. Experiment with different products that contain a diverse array of nutrients. Remember that water is indispensable to your body's processes and you need at least 6 to 8 glasses of fluid a day.

Diet and health

If you 'feel' that your body is suffering, try the following general guidelines that are promoted by many health authorities around the world. They recommend that you avoid excess sugar, fatty foods, salt, excessive levels of protein, alcohol, highly processed food and caffeine.

Most of us consume too much of the above, and often suffer problems later in life. Start now and modify your consumption. Substitute fresh, wholesome, natural fruit, vegetables and cereals. Aim to spend twice as much at the greengrocer's and half as much in the supermarket!

See the Vitamins and minerals table on pages 48 and 49 to learn how vitamins and minerals perform in your body.

Protecting food quality

Always buy the freshest, highest quality food you can afford. When preparing, cooking and storing food, always think about the fragile vitamins and minerals in cell juices and how to protect them. You have just paid a lot of money for them. Try to buy small amounts of very fresh fruit and vegetables every two to three days.

Wash and cut fruit and vegetables just before use. Cook whole if possible to capture the goodness. Steaming, stir-frying and other fast methods of cooking are preferable as they ensure minimum vitamin loss. Eat before your food cools, chewing well to break up cell walls. Longer cooking in soups, stews and casseroles will release more minerals into the fluid.

tip

Brief yourself on the full range of skin foods by consulting our vitamins and minerals table, page 48. Vitamin A and vitamin E are very important for healing skin and eyes and for offsetting pollution. The B vitamins – B2, B3 and B6 assist. Vitamin C is a detoxifier. Copper, iron and zinc are all important minerals.

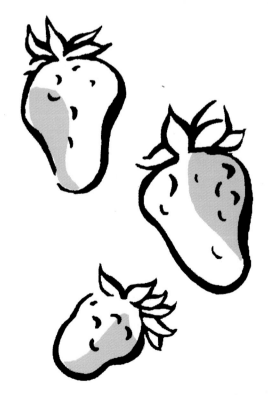

Glossary

ANTIBODY	neutralizes foreign protein
ANTIOXIDANT	protects from toxic substances
ASTRINGENT	contracts skin
BACTERIA	simple microscopic organisms
BETACAROTENE	yellow pigment (vitamin A)
CANDIDA	fungal infection
CAPILLARIES	tiny blood vessels
CHEMOTHERAPY	chemical treatment of disease
COMPRESS	soft cloth pad, often cotton
DERMIS	inner skin layer
EFFLEURAGE	gentle massage stroke
EPIDERMIS	outer skin layer
EXPECTORANT	releases phlegm, mucus
FATTY ACID	component of fats, oils
FIBROUS TRAP	filters lymph
HAEMOGLOBIN	red pigment in blood
HAIR FOLLICLE	produces hair shaft
HENNA	natural plant dye, treatment
HORMONE	complex molecule controlling body processes
KERATIN	protein in hair and nails
LYMPH	colourless fluid surrounding cells
LYMPH NODE	site of waste breakdown
LYMPHATIC SYSTEM	cleans body of wastes
NADI SYSTEM	energy network underlying nerves
pH BALANCE	measure of acidity/alkalinity
SEBUM	waxy oil in skin
SHIATSU	Eastern energy-flow massage
SITZ BATH	curative hip bath
SOLUBLE FIBRE	plant fibre dissolving in water
THYROID	hormone centre in throat
TONIC	invigorating medicine
TOXINS	wastes produced by cells
VACCINE	inoculation against disease

Index